Palliative Care
in Severe Dementia
in association with *Nursing and Residential Care*

i

Palliative Care
in Severe Dementia

in association with *Nursing and Residential Care*

edited by

Julian C Hughes

QUAY
BOOKS

A division of MA Healthcare Ltd

Quay Books Division, MA Healthcare Ltd, St Jude's Church, Dulwich Road,
London SE24 0PB

British Library Cataloguing-in-Publication Data
A catalogue record is available for this book

© MA Healthcare Limited 2006
ISBN 1 85642 265 8

Printed in the UK by Bath Press, Lower Bristol Road, Bath B2 3BL, UK

Contents

List of contributors

Clive Baldwin is Senior Lecturer at Bradford Dementia Group, University of Bradford. He was previously a Research Fellow at The Oxford Centre for Ethics and Communication in Health Care Practice (The Ethox Centre).

Audrey Ball was previously Catholic Chaplain for Newcastle City Health NHS Trust, based at St Nicholas Hospital, Gosforth, Newcastle upon Tyne.

Clive Ballard is Professor of Age Related Disorders at the Institute of Psychiatry and King's College, London. He is also Director of Research at the Alzheimer's Society. He was previously Professor of Old Age Psychiatry in the University of Newcastle.

Lynne Corner is a Research Associate at the Centre for Health Services Research and Institute for Ageing and Health at the University of Newcastle, where she previously held an Alzheimer's Society Research Fellowship.

Leslie Dinning is a full time Chaplain with Newcastle, North Tyneside and Northumberland NHS Mental Health Trust and a Methodist Local Preacher.

Simon Douglas is a Clinical Research Nurse in the Wolfson Research Centre, Institute for Ageing and Health, University of Newcastle.

Philip Dove is a Staff Nurse at Ashgrove Nursing Home, Newcastle, North Tyneside and Northumberland Mental Health NHS Trust.

Debra Harris was previously Clinical Team Leader at Ashgrove Nursing Home, Newcastle, North Tyneside and Northumberland Mental Health NHS Trust.

Kathleen Hedley was (until the summer of 2005) Home Manager at Ashgrove Nursing Home, Newcastle, North Tyneside and Northumberland Mental Health NHS Trust.

Julian C Hughes is a Consultant in Old Age Psychiatry in Northumbria Healthcare NHS Trust and an Honorary Clinical Senior Lecturer in the University of Newcastle. He was a consultant at Newcastle General Hospital with responsibility for Ashgrove Nursing Home between 1999 and 2004.

Lisa Hulford is a Staff Nurse at Ashgrove Nursing Home, Newcastle, North Tyneside and Northumberland Mental Health NHS Trust.

Margaret E Huntley is a Clinical Team Leader at Ashgrove Nursing Home, Newcastle, North Tyneside and Northumberland Mental Health NHS Trust.

Ian James is a Consultant Clinical Psychologist at Newcastle General Hospital, employed by Newcastle, North Tyneside and Northumberland Mental Health NHS Trust.

Claud Regnard is a Consultant in Palliative Medicine, St. Oswald's Hospice, Newcastle City Hospitals NHS Trust and Northgate and Prudhoe NHS Trust.

Louise Robinson is a general practitioner and Clinical Senior Lecturer in dementia and ageing research, Centre for Health Services Research, University of Newcastle.

Jill Summersall is a Specialist Speech and Language Therapist in Old Age Psychiatry, working in the Newcastle, North Tyneside and Northumberland Mental Health NHS Trust.

Sheila Wight is a Specialist Speech and Language Therapist in Old Age Psychiatry, working in the Newcastle, North Tyneside and Northumberland Mental Health NHS Trust.

Disclaimer

The views expressed in this book are entirely personal to the authors and cannot be taken to reflect the opinions of the employing Trusts or other organizations. The case histories, although based on reality, are fictional. Every effort has been made to ensure that details of drugs and drug dosages are accurate, but no guarantee can be given and readers are urged to check local, contemporaneous, authoritative sources before any drugs are prescribed. Similarly, psychosocial interventions should only be given by properly trained and registered practitioners.

Dedication

This work is dedicated to the present and past residents, their families, carers and all the staff in Ashgrove Nursing Home, Gosforth, Newcastle upon Tyne.

Preface

Julian C Hughes

This book stems from practice, from the experience of providing care to people with severe dementia. The roots of our interests and concerns are probably very deep. Suffice to say that when I took up a consultant post at Newcastle General Hospital in 1999, I was delighted to find myself involved with Ashgrove Nursing Home.

In health and social service jargon, this is an Elderly Severely Mentally Infirm (ESMI) unit. It would also be called a National Health Service (NHS) continuing care unit, which sounds rather dry. What I found was a home with staff dedicated to the care of people with severe dementia. Over the course of five years I observed the senior nurse, Kathy Hedley, who became the manager, lead the staff through some difficult times, with staff shortages, bureaucratic hassles and bits of the (new) building falling down. More than this, however, I was instantly struck by Kathy's commitment to a palliative care approach. For her, Ashgrove was a hospice for people with dementia. This philosophy is fleshed out in the first two chapters of this book.

As time went on, I realized that among us there was a body of knowledge and expertise that it was not easy to find recorded in one place. When I say 'among us', I mean among the nursing staff; but I also include all those other people who contributed to the care of the residents in the home. Claud Regnard was known, at times, to visit the home over a weekend if urgent advice on palliative care were needed. (Of course, he will deny there is anything extraordinary in this!) Our psychology colleagues (represented in this volume by Ian James) were at hand to give advice on behavioural issues. We benefited hugely from the expert suggestions about swallowing difficulties provided by the speech and language therapists, such as Jill Summersall and Sheila Wight. The home was well served by two general practitioners, who provided the day-to-day health care for the residents. Perhaps the person I came across most often, apart from the nursing staff, was Les Dinning, the chaplain, whose services to the residents – and in particular to their family carers – was greatly appreciated, as was the work of others in the chaplaincy team, such as Audrey Ball.

This litany only includes those whose names appear elsewhere in this book. But this is not to say that the knowledge and expertise was not more widely spread. It simply reflects my inability to record the names of all those who must contribute to the wellbeing of people with severe dementia. I have not mentioned the dentist, the podiatrist, the pharmacist, the physiotherapist, the hairdresser, etc. I should also record that my responsibilities within Ashgrove were shared with Dr Ann Scully until 2003.

There is a sense in which trying to make a book serve as a repository of knowledge and experience around palliative care in dementia is a futile task. I remember discussing a particular resident with a nurse during a review meeting. The nurse had already painted the picture of the person as being completely dependent with severe dementia, but he went on to suggest that you could always tell the resident's mood. For the sake of interest, given that I was aware the resident had no means of verbal communication, I asked how the nurse could tell a good from a bad mood. I suspect the nurse thought I was completely naïve, but he went on to list subtle and not so subtle gestures, movements, expressions, behaviours and grimaces that might indicate this or that feeling. A book cannot capture well enough the expertise that depends upon the relationships built up over time between the carer and the cared for. Certainly nothing in this book captures adequately the importance of the commitment of the staff in homes such as Ashgrove.

None of us would suggest, I think, despite its largely good local reputation, that Ashgrove was any better than similar homes. In writing this book, we have not intended to suggest that we have more expertise in this field than any others up and down the country. Newcastle, however, has always been a centre of expertise as far as research on dementia goes. We have been able to call upon some of this expertise in writing this book. Simon Douglas and Clive Ballard (before he went to London) from the Institute for Ageing and Health, and Lynne Corner and Louise Robinson from the Centre for Health Services Research, all within the University of Newcastle, have made valuable contributions.

The only 'outsider' was Clive Baldwin, now with the Bradford Dementia Group in the University of Bradford. Clive and I have known each other since he worked in the Ethox Centre in the University of Oxford (with Tony Hope, Robin Jacoby and Sue Ziebland), where he was the main researcher on a project funded by the Alzheimer's Society to look at the ethical issues that arise for family carers of people with dementia. My original intention was to try to involve family carers from Ashgrove in the writing of this book. But this proved difficult, in part I think because they were too raw from their experiences and too burdened already. Clive's deep understanding of the issues facing family carers, therefore, was invaluable. One of the striking things at Ashgrove, as elsewhere, has been the continuing involvement of family carers – who at one and the same time can be both challenging and supportive. It is our privilege to know them at a very difficult time in their lives.

I owe a large debt of gratitude to all of the contributors to this book, who put up with a lot of editorial interference. I am particularly grateful to the nurses – Debbie, Kathy, Lisa, Margaret and Philip – who contributed; but I am also grateful to the other nurses in Ashgrove from whom I have learnt much over the years. It was always a pleasure and an inspiration.

The idea for the series of articles that appeared in *Nursing and Residential Care* in 2004, which now form this book, was concocted with the editor of that journal, Charlotte Dennis-Jones. Towards the end of the year Caroline Finucane took over as editor. Charlotte and Caroline have both been the easiest, most efficient and kind people to work with. They took my last-minuteness and panicky changes in their stride. In a similar way, the initial discussions about the book were conducted with Binkie Mais, who was always encouraging; but Helena Raeside has shouldered the burden of turning our incoherent amendments into something more professional. I am also grateful to Jessica Anderson for her efficient and helpful work producing the proofs of the book. Closer to home, Agnes Muse has provided much needed secretarial support with her usual good humour and coffee. Meanwhile, at home, Anne, Olli, Emma and Luke have put up with monthly angst, as the series appeared, with lashings of benign understanding. And Luke produced *Figure 11.1*. I am hugely grateful to them all.

I said above that, when the ideas behind this book were being formulated, it was difficult to find a single place with the requisite knowledge and expertise recorded. I soon discovered, however, another work that contains years of scholarship from the USA in this field. At several points we have referred to the book by Volicer and Hurley (1998). Their book has been an inspiration. This book provides a different approach and aims at a slightly different audience. In particular, we present a UK perspective.

One of the further benefits to me in editing this book is to have become acquainted with Ladislav Volicer, who must be regarded as the pioneer of palliative care in dementia. Exactly how things might develop in this field in the UK is a moot point, but my thoughts have certainly been stimulated by discussions with various friends and colleagues in Newcastle and further afield (Hughes et al, 2005). I hope this modest work will go some way towards encouraging the conversations that are already occurring. Certainly it is the hope of all concerned that the quality of care for people with severe dementia should improve.

References

Hughes JC, Robinson L, Volicer L (2005) Specialist palliative care in dementia. *Br Med J* **330**: 57-8

Volicer L, Hurley A (eds) (1998) *Hospice Care for Patients with Advanced Progressive Dementia*. Springer, New York

Chapter 1

The practice and philosophy of palliative care in dementia

Julian C Hughes, Kathleen Hedley, Debra Harris

Palliative care for people with severe dementia: what does it involve? In this chapter, we shall consider what constitutes palliative care. We shall then ask: is this approach relevant to people with severe dementia? Our answer will be that not only is it relevant, but also it provides an ethical way to approach the care of people with severe dementia (Purtilo and ten Have, 2004).

What is palliative care?

In 1967, Dame Cicely Saunders founded St Christopher's Hospice in London. From this beginning the hospice movement has grown hugely throughout the world. Hospices are the most public manifestation of palliative care, which is defined as:

> *'The active total care of patients whose disease is not responsive to curative treatment. Control of pain, of other symptoms, and of psychological, social and spiritual problems is paramount.' (World Health Organization, 1990)*

According to this definition, palliative care:

- Affirms life and regards dying as a normal process so that death should neither be hastened nor postponed
- Provides relief from distressing symptoms
- Integrates the psychological, social and spiritual aspects of care
- Offers support to dying people to live as actively as possible until death
- Offers support to families coping with the person's illness and their bereavement (Sidell et al, 2000).

The hospice movement has encouraged a general acceptance of these

---

Table 1.1: Definitions

Palliative care approach
- Promotes physical and psychosocial wellbeing
- Integral to all clinical practice whatever the illness
- Informed by principles of palliative care
- Supported by specialist palliative care

Palliative interventions
- Non-curative treatments aimed at controlling distressing symptoms and improving a person's quality of life

Specialist palliative care
- Services with palliative care as core speciality
- Provided directly through specialist service or indirectly through patient's current health team
- Multidisciplinary, providing physical, psychological, social and spiritual support

---

principles in routine clinical practice. In addition, hospices provide centres of expertise for the control of pain in advanced cancer.

Palliative care forms a spectrum (*Table 1.1*) (Addington-Hall, 1998). At one end lies supportive (palliative) care which makes use of the principles outlined above; while at the other, specialist palliative care concentrates on complex cases. Between these two lie palliative interventions such as radiotherapy, chemotherapy, and anaesthetic or surgical techniques, which are normally given by health-care professionals other than palliative care specialists.

It would be complacent to assume that the principles of palliative care are put into practice everywhere. Nevertheless, the approach is potentially available throughout the UK and in many parts of the world. It is still the case, however, that it has mainly focused on cancer. Issues around extending palliative care to non-cancer patients are complex and moves in this direction face a number of possible barriers, including (Field and Addington-Hall, 2000):

- A lack of skills among specialist palliative care experts in the care of non-cancer patients
- Difficulties surrounding the identification of patients for such services
- Concern over the acceptability of such services for non-cancer patients
- Resource implications
- Vested interests.

Nevertheless, such barriers should not be regarded as insurmountable (Simard and Volicer, 1998). Field and Addington-Hall (2000) concluded:

'Although there have been almost no evaluations of specialist palliative care provision for patients who die from causes other than cancer, there is now convincing evidence that conventional care

alone is not meeting the needs of such patients. Thus, what is not in doubt is that the status quo is unacceptable.'

The question is: In what ways is palliative care (broadly understood) relevant to the care of people with severe dementia?

Palliative care approach

The palliative care approach should be integral to all clinical practice involving chronic, terminal disease. Therefore by definition it is entirely suited to the care of people with advanced dementia (Black and Jolley, 1990). The underpinning principles are as follows (Addington-Hall, 1998):

- A focus on quality of life, including good symptom control
- A 'whole person' approach
- Care that encompasses not solely the person with the life-threatening disease but also those who matter to him or her
- Respect for the person's autonomy
- An emphasis on open and sensitive communication which extends to patients, informal carers and colleagues.

Quality of life

In severe dementia quality of life is circumscribed. When a person can no longer communicate verbally, is reliant on others for all personal care and has become immobile, it can be difficult to see what quality of life remains. However, those who work closely with people in the severe stages of dementia will be able to point to numerous ways in which the person demonstrates individuality. In particular, carers will be aware of when the person with dementia is distressed or calm, content or discontent.

The aim of good quality care is to maximize quality of life. One consequence is that this takes precedence over quantity of life. Sheer survival is not an aim of palliative care. In all of these respects, the focus on quality of life is highly relevant to work with people with severe dementia. The emphasis should be on good nursing (Watson, 1994):

'In the case of dementia, active treatment can effectively be replaced by intensive nursing and comfort measures.'

Issues around quality of life are discussed further in Chapter 8. However, given that what makes up quality of life is diverse for individuals, maintaining it will be a multidisciplinary endeavour that will give rise to social, emotional and spiritual issues for patients, families and professional carers (Kearney, 1992).

The holistic view

This leads us to consider the person as a 'whole'. The person, even in severe dementia, can be considered as a situated embodied agent (Hughes, 2001). As an agent, the person can still show signs of distress (e.g. by grimaces or groans) which should be detected by carers. The 'agentive' nature will entail the possibility of fears concerning increased dependency, isolation and the maintenance of privacy and dignity.

The person's embodied nature means that his or her physical needs require careful attention. In dementia this will, as elsewhere in palliative care, mean attention to pain relief; similarly, it will include mouth care, skin care, help with feeding, moving and toileting, with alertness to the risks of choking, constipation, falls and infections.

The person is also situated in numerous contexts, not least of which is a personal history without which he or she will not be fully understood. The person might also be situated in a cultural background different to that of the carers, but towards which they must be sensitive. The person is situated in a spiritual context too, whether or not this involves adherence to a specific religious faith. The importance of the spiritual dimension means that it should be an essential component of nursing practice (Govier, 2000). (Spiritual care is considered again in Chapter 12.) The holistic view, therefore, is essential to good quality care in severe dementia.

Family and friends

Crucially, the person is situated in a context of family and friends, so care of the person with dementia entails care of those that he or she loves. Of course, not everyone that we look after has family or friends, but then it becomes all the more important that the human environment we provide should be enhancing and not detracting.

The familial context will be relevant at all stages of dementia, but (arguably) it becomes more so as the illness progresses. In the later stages of dementia, family or close friends appropriately become the main focus for decision-making in the person's best interests. The sort of difficult decisions that face family carers are portrayed in Chapter 9. Carers' physical, psychological, social and spiritual needs must also be considered even while the interests of the person with dementia remain paramount.

Relatives, especially when they are themselves older, might suffer ill health, fatigue, immobility or physical symptoms associated with stress. This might limit their ability to visit the person they have previously cared for. They will also tend to have anxieties about the health of the person with dementia, which may be associated with fears about his or her death. Alternatively, they might worry about dying first. Feelings of guilt on the part of close family carers are common when the person with dementia has been placed in a long-term home. Guilt might be associated with depression. On the other hand, such anxieties might manifest themselves by way of critical comments directed at the staff of the home.

Socially, the family carer may feel isolated once the person with severe dementia is in a home. Spending long hours visiting might lead to other areas of social life being neglected, and after the person's death the one-time carers might find themselves bereft of the social stimulation visiting the home once provided. The social losses might also include financial strains as well as the loss of a friend and perhaps sexual partner.

From the spiritual perspective, there may be a loss of faith or simply a feeling of no longer belonging in the world. In short, for families and friends, dementia becomes a protracted, lingering bereavement. The palliative care approach takes family and friends seriously and is, therefore, entirely apt for dementia care.

Autonomy

In cancer care, respect for autonomy will usually mean discussing treatment options (including the location of treatment) with the patient. In severe dementia this is usually not possible. One obvious way to respect autonomy is to take heed of the person's advance directive, or 'living will'. However, very few people with dementia in the UK have such documents at present. As long as the advance directive is clearly established, applicable to current circumstances and made without undue pressure, it has a legal basis. But it is more correctly referred to as an 'advance refusal of treatment', since patients cannot insist on particular treatments, even if they can refuse them.

There are concerns about advance directives. Whether they will be applicable to the person's current circumstances will depend on whether the person has correctly foreseen what those circumstances might be like. The person with dementia, who nevertheless seems content, might be the person who once regarded dementia as the condition most to dread. At a deeper philosophical level, questions have been raised about whether he or she is the same person as the person before the onset of dementia who made the advance refusal (Hope, 1995).

However, perhaps a more immediate philosophical and practical challenge comes from simply trying to understand what autonomy means in individual cases. For a long while it has been regarded as the main principle of medical ethics, but it is by no means a straightforward notion (Collopy, 1988). In severe dementia particularly, respecting a person's autonomy will require not only attention to past wishes, but also an awareness of the person's current physical, psychological, social and spiritual circumstances. This will bring into play all of the aspects of palliative care already mentioned, including the involvement of family and other close carers. It also necessitates thought about communication.

Communication

Communication becomes difficult when patients may have severe expressive and receptive problems. Loss of concentration and poor memory add to these difficulties. However, emotional receptivity and meaning do not inevitably disappear even in severe dementia, and attempts to communicate should persist (Sabat, 2001). Tactile communication, feeding, or simply 'being with', are also means of conveying emotional tone.

Communication with the family is vital. Information needs to be provided sensitively and appropriately. It occurs over time, with a need for repetition and pacing. Ordinary communication is not entirely disease-focused; chatting and joking can help to foster a relaxed environment (Dean, 2002).

Communication between members of the care team needs to be effective, open and honest to ensure the holistic approach is maintained consistently. The physical and psychological demands of this type of nursing, along with the spiritual questions it raises, mean that staff should be appropriately supported within teams and by management.

The case study below is a surprising way, perhaps, to conclude this section, but not if the palliative care approach is taken seriously. The potential surprise is that it demonstrates the importance of good communication with people with dementia, even where this might seem problematic. It is also potentially surprising because when we talk of bereavement in connection with dementia, we are usually thinking of the bereaved carers. However, this case study demonstrates the relevance of thinking broadly about the person's quality of life, taking symptoms seriously, involving important others, respecting the person's autonomy and being sensitive in communication.

Case study: Arnold's grief

At the time of his wife's death, Arnold had only been in an elderly severely mentally infirm (ESMI) nursing home for a short while. But Elsie, his wife, had made it plain that she did not wish her husband to be informed about her cancer. Still, when she died his son asked a nurse to inform Arnold immediately.

Arnold's dementia left him with little language and, on being told, he showed no obvious emotional upset but simply smiled and spoke incoherent words. When the family arrived, Arnold continued to show no obvious response to the news, although they talked to him for some while about Elsie's death. The family were themselves shocked by their bereavement and anxious about the effects on Arnold. They, too, needed support.

Arnold could not attend the funeral but a short service was put on by the chaplain, during which Arnold remained outwardly unmoved. However, once the service was over and the family had returned to their busy lives, Arnold became more overtly upset and anxious. Although the cause of his anxiety and aggression was not immediately obvious it became clearer that he was calling Elsie's name at times of agitation. The main nurse, who throughout this time had been intimately involved with Arnold's care, spent much time with him, talking gently to him about Elsie and her death. His anxiety could sometimes be calmed by a hug but the emotional involvement with him was also difficult for the nurse.

On occasions, when the family returned, Arnold would appear aggressive towards them. It was surmised that he – in some sense – blamed them for not bringing Elsie to see him. Although the nurse had a good relationship with Arnold, his anxiety and agitation were persisting.

Following a case review, Arnold's consultant psychiatrist prescribed an antidepressant and it was agreed that the clinical psychologist should be involved. Arnold seemed stuck in the work of grief. Aromatherapy was used via a diffuser and by massage. Gradually the time spent with Arnold seemed to be calming him. The psychologist also suggested that a memory box, containing items reminiscent of Elsie, should be made up and used to encourage memories and talk of her and of their life together. The memory box was used by the family as well as by the main nurse, but always tentatively in case Arnold was not in a receptive mood. Generally, however, Arnold appeared happier when talking, albeit incoherently, about items in the box. He continued to express anxiety and sadness but the calmer periods were longer. He seemed to value the time spent with his main nurse and to enjoy more the visits from the family.

Palliative versus person-centred care

Many people working in the field of dementia care will be more familiar with a paradigm other than that of palliative care. Person-centred care, intimately linked with the name of the late Tom Kitwood, puts the person with dementia first (Kitwood, 1997).

Proponents of Kitwood's approach might look askance at the idea that people with dementia should be regarded in the same light as people with terminal cancer. First, however, palliative care is not simply a matter of terminal

Table 1.2: Psychological needs of people with dementia and aspects of palliative care		
Psychological needs (Kitwood, 1997)	WHO definition of palliative care (WHO, 1990)	Aspects of the palliative care approach (Addington-Hall,1998)
Attachment	Support to person and family	Importance of sensitive communication
Comfort	Symptom control	Quality of life
Identity	Integration of psychological, social and spiritual aspects	Whole person approach
Occupation	Affirmation of life	Respect for autonomy
Inclusion	Support to person and family	Care of person and family

care. The approach stresses a broader attitude towards life; it is not just about dying well, but about living well until the point of death. Second, it follows that palliative care, with its emphasis on quality of life, should not be a philosophy of 'no hope'. In fact it challenges the traditional type of care given to people with severe dementia in much the same way as person-centred dementia care. A holistic view which aims to respect a person's autonomy and support his or her quality of life will in many cases require a change in attitudes, better training and more appropriate resources.

Third, it might be argued that Kitwood's philosophy should be applied to the mild to moderate stages of dementia, while the palliative care approach should be used in severe dementia. But this would be wrong. *Table 1.2* shows what Kitwood (1997) regarded as the main psychological needs of people with dementia. Juxtaposed are the elements of the WHO's definition and the aspects of the palliative care approach we have been discussing so far. The extent of the matching of the paradigms is clear and for one reason: they are motivated by a concern for the person. Specifically, they are motivated by the concern that the person should not be 'written off' by a diagnosis.

In Kitwood's terms, 'attachment' reflects the need for secure bonds with family and carers; 'comfort' includes the relief of pain but also suggests closeness and tenderness; 'identity' requires a narrative, which may be known by others; 'occupation' means being involved in the process of life and may, again, depend on those around the person; 'inclusion' suggests the need to have our social standing as persons recognized.

One interesting feature of *Table 1.2* is the way in which Kitwood's psychological needs bring in aspects of a physical and social nature. The reason for this stems from the notion of the person discussed above, as a situated-embodied-agent, which inherently involves physical, psychological and social aspects in a way that allows one to spill over into another. Thus, being physically unwell affects mood and social interactions, while being in solitary confinement would affect mental state.

Furthermore, these aspects of personhood are not the only ones – there may be cultural or historical aspects. But for Kitwood the overarching need is for love. The human need for interconnectedness is at the heart of good nursing, whether as part of the palliative care approach or as an integral aspect of person-centred care.

Conclusion

We have outlined what constitutes palliative care and have shown how it is relevant to people with severe dementia (Wilson et al, 1996). We have not lingered over terminal care in advanced dementia, although there is evidence that this is inadequate (Lloyd-Williams, 1996). Nor have we delved into what are called 'palliative interventions' in *Table 1.1*, which in severe dementia would include psychopharmacological and psychosocial or behavioural therapy. These topics, along with further exploration of some of the issues raised here, will be covered in other chapters.

We have shown that the palliative care approach can be mapped onto person-centred care in a way that would be beneficial to those with severe dementia. An underlying assumption of person-centred care is that personhood is, in part, a function of the individual's situatedness. That is, the person is a person among others. Hence, the attitudes and actions of others can either enhance or diminish the standing of the individual.

Person-centred care and palliative care give a moral significance to the importance of the person, whether or not he or she has dementia, right up to the point of death. Given, therefore, the ethical case in favour of treating people with dementia as persons in the fullest possible sense (Post, 2000), the argument that there is an ethical imperative to deliver palliative care in severe dementia is easily won.

References

Addington-Hall J (1998) *Reaching Out: Specialist Palliative Care for Adults with Non-Malignant Disease*. Occasional Paper 14. National Council for Hospice and Specialist Palliative Care Services, London: 8

Black D, Jolley D (1990) Slow euthanasia? The deaths of psychogeriatric patients. *Br*

Med J **300**(6735): 1321–3

Collopy BJ (1988) Autonomy in long-term care: some crucial distinctions. *Gerontologist* **28**(3suppl): 10–7

Dean A (2002) Talking to dying patients of their hopes and needs. *Nurs Times* **98**(43): 34–5

Field D, Addington-Hall J (2000) Extending specialist palliative care to all? In: Dickenson D, Johnson M, Katz JS (eds) *Death, Dying and Bereavement*. Open University and Sage, London: 91–106

Govier I (2000) Spiritual care in nursing: a systematic approach. *Nurs Stand* **14**(17): 32–6

Hope T (1995) Personal identity and psychiatric illness. In: Griffiths AP (ed) *Philosophy, Psychology and Psychiatry*. Cambridge University Press, Cambridge: 131–43

Hughes JC (2001) Views of the person with dementia. *J Med Ethics* **27**(2): 86–91

Kearney M (1992) Palliative medicine – just another specialty. *Palliat Med* **6**: 39–46

Kitwood T (1997) *Dementia Reconsidered: The Person Comes First*. Open University Press, Buckingham and Philadelphia

Lloyd-Williams M (1996) An audit of palliative care in dementia. *Eur J Cancer Care* **5**(1): 53–5

Post SG (2000) *The Moral Challenge of Alzheimer's Disease: Ethical Issues from Diagnosis to Dying*. 2nd edn. Johns Hopkins University Press, Baltimore

Purtilo RB, ten Have HAMJ (eds) (2004) *Ethical Foundations of Palliative Care for Alzheimer's Disease*. Johns Hopkins University Press, Baltimore.

Sabat SR (2001) *The Experience of Alzheimer's Disease: Life Through a Tangled Veil*. Blackwell, Oxford

Sidell M, Katz JS, Komaromy C (2000) The case for palliative care in residential and nursing homes. In: Dickenson D, Johnson M, Katz JS (eds) *Death, Dying and Bereavement*. Open University and Sage, London: 107–21

Simard J, Volicer L (1998) Barriers to providing hospice care for people with dementia. In: Volicer L, Hurley A (eds) *Hospice Care for Patients with Advanced Progressive Dementia*. Springer, New York: 231–46

Watson R (1994) Towards a compassionate model of care. *J Dementia Care* **2**(6) 18–19

Wilson SA, Kovach CR, Stearns SA (1996) Hospice concepts in the care for end-stage dementia. *Geriatr Nurs* **17**(1): 6–10

World Health Organization (1990) *Technical Report Series 804*. World Health Organization, Geneva

Key points

- Palliative care involves considering quality of life (including symptom control), a holistic view of the person, concern for the person's family and friends, respect for autonomy and good communication.

- Each of these aspects of care is relevant to the care of people with severe dementia.

- Indeed, the palliative care approach and person-centred dementia care, although different paradigms, are motivated by the same concern for the person.

- Moreover, there is an ethical imperative to the need for a broad-based and challenging conception of care for those with severe dementia.

- Palliative care provides a hopeful model for the care of people with severe dementia.

Chapter 2

Aspects of holistic terminal care in severe dementia

Kathleen Hedley, Julian C Hughes

One of the guiding principles of palliative care is that, as well as providing an integrated approach to the care of the dying, families should be helped to cope with the person's illness and their own bereavement. Using a case study, we shall discuss what 'holistic' means in practical terms and its underlying ethical basis. Thus, in this chapter, we shall flesh out some of the discussion in Chapter 1.

It is of interest that, in no part of Standard 7 (which concerns mental health and deals with dementia) of the National Service Framework (NSF) for Older People (Department of Health, 2001) is there a mention of palliative care. It is true that there is passing reference to the need for supportive and palliative care in Standard 2, which relates to person-centred care – *Table 2.1* records the principles commended in the NSF. But the failure to mention palliative care, in its discussion of the services required for dementia, is a regrettable oversight.

Nevertheless, the principles set out in *Table 2.1* can be applied to the care of people with severe dementia. The interesting thing to note is that, in the terminal phases of dementia, some of the principles are just as applicable to the informal carer as they are to the person with dementia. That is the feature of holistic care to be highlighted in this chapter: holism not only means a broad approach to the person with dementia, it also entails recognition of the context of relationships in which the person is embedded.

Table 2.1: End-of-life care

- Information and communication
- Control of painful and other distressing symptoms
- Rehabilitation and support as health declines
- Social care
- Spiritual care
- Complementary therapies
- Psychological care
- Bereavement support

The case study: Father and son

The case of Ernie and his son, Len, helps to focus attention on the unit of care.

Case study: Ernie and his son

Ernie was an 83-year-old resident in long-term care with a 7-year history of Alzheimer's disease. He was now immobile, physically very frail, thin and increasingly susceptible to infections. In the last weeks of his life he deteriorated rapidly. He was still able to sit in the lounge with other residents, although his posture became foetal. This affected his feeding and drinking: it became almost impossible to position him suitably.

After a discussion between the doctor and Ernie's key worker, liquid food supplements where prescribed. Initially, with patience and the careful use of a feeding cup, this proved quite successful.

For some time Ernie had suffered from recurring chest infections. His posture exacerbated this tendency since it impeded the drainage of fluid from his chest and both his cough and swallowing reflexes were impaired. Amoxicillin tended to deal with minor chest infections, but in the week before his death Ernie deteriorated rapidly with a diagnosis of bronchopneumonia.

His son, Len, who was a regular visitor, met with Ernie's key worker and consultant. They discussed Ernie's physical condition and answered Len's questions about his father's prognosis and management. The difficult issue of artificial hydration was discussed and the pros and cons of the various procedures (subcutaneous or intravenous drip, naso-gastric tube or percutaneous endoscopic gastrostomy – i.e. a feeding tube placed straight through the abdominal wall into the stomach) were fully explained. Len asked that his father should be kept comfortable and pain-free. His general inclination to avoid invasive therapies was accepted by the team and entered into Ernie's medical and nursing notes. It was agreed, however, that aromatherapy hand massage, as a gentle means of contact, should be provided by the member of staff trained in this technique, or by Len if he wished.

Ernie appeared to be nearing death. He was accepting very little fluid and was being nursed in bed. He was drifting in and out of consciousness. The decision was made with the involvement of Len to stop regular medication and to treat Ernie purely palliatively.

Good companions

Reassessment of Ernie's physical condition was carried out, which involved assessment of his skin integrity. Moving and handling were kept to a minimum with the help of a pressure-relieving mattress. Ernie was incontinent of both faeces and urine. Since urine output was minimal, it was not thought appropriate to use a catheter. Incontinence pads were used, although this then necessitated occasional movement.

Len was now staying at the home 24 hours a day, sleeping in the visitor's room. The nurses were aware of the stress he was under. As the days passed, every effort was made to make time to talk to him and to listen as he spoke about his memories and the good times he had enjoyed with his father when he was growing up. They were very close, since his mother had died when he was young and Len had never married. The home chaplain became involved and visited regularly to lend spiritual support and to spend time with them both. Len's many friends also visited with offers of help – their visits were encouraged by the home as a way to ease Len's feelings of isolation.

One evening, however, while talking to night staff, he mentioned how much he missed his dog and how concerned he was about her. His dog, Carrie, had previously come to the home whenever Len visited his father and was spoilt by staff and residents alike. The next day arrangements were made for Carrie to stay too. This gave Len another focus, much comfort, and a distraction from the ordeal of watching his father die.

Palliative work

Ernie by this time was beginning to suffer from breathlessness (dyspnoea), probably related to his bronchopneumonia. This symptom was managed by ensuring that he was positioned as upright as possible, and that the room was well ventilated. At the same time Len was reassured that, although the symptom was seemingly distressing for Ernie, it could be tended to by this fairly simple means and, indeed, it did ease considerably. Ernie himself continued to drift in and out of consciousness.

Ernie had now developed a noisy chest on account of the build-up of secretions on his lungs which he was too weak to clear himself. His son, Len, found this 'death-rattle' particularly distressing. So, after further discussions within the multidisciplinary team, hyoscine hydrobromide was prescribed as a patch (to obviate the need for Ernie to swallow).

From the onset of Ernie's deterioration, oral hygiene was incorporated into his care plan. Chips of ice were used to moisten his mouth and Vaseline used to keep his lips moist. Len offered ice chips when he thought Ernie appeared parched. Len was also encouraged, when he wanted, to help with his father's personal hygiene. Therefore in various ways Len was made to feel a part of the process and not a helpless bystander.

Ernie had now been near to death for 5 days. The question of hydration again arose within the team, with some staff beginning to worry that he had been without fluids for too long. The concerns were shared with Len, who reiterated his original inclination to avoid invasive treatment. The original decision was reaffirmed; to carry on with purely palliative treatment.

Closing moments

At this point, although unconscious, the nursing team felt that during interventions Ernie appeared to wince slightly. The doctor was consulted and diamorphine hydrochloride was prescribed (to be administered by subcutaneous injection at 5mg every 4 hours).

Everyone agreed that Ernie had seemed pain-free up until this time and the idea that he was now suffering pain was unacceptable. Len was in agreement with this, but the realization that his father needed morphine brought home to him the reality of his father's imminent death. He was able to discuss this with staff and the chaplain who continued to visit. Before Ernie could receive any Diamorphine, however, he died peacefully one evening with his son and staff at his bedside.

After his father's death, Len stayed with his body for some while, until the on-call doctor certified the death. Len then sat with staff reminiscing. The next day he returned to sort out practical matters. Members of staff attended the funeral and Len continued to visit the home from time to time in the weeks and months after Ernie's death, but gradually his visits tailed off. On the occasion of the first anniversary of his father's death, however, Len visited again. He was emotional, but pleased to see the members of staff who had known his father. He left knowing that he could contact the home at any time.

Health workers typically say that their duty of care is to the patient. In terminal care, however, it is difficult to escape the fact that people are located in a context of care which involves others. Therefore, holistic terminal care inevitably means the care of the whole family; or, at least, those who are engaged with the person who is ill. Usually this involves the family but it may include 'significant others'. Not all those engaged with a dying person will want to receive the attentions of professionals. But in caring for the dying person, professionals must at least be open to the needs of these others.

Information and communication

Communication with people with severe dementia becomes difficult but it is a means of contributing to their wellbeing (Kitwood, 1997). Ernie required both verbal and non-verbal reassurance when he was being re-positioned. In addition, throughout the terminal phase of his father's illness, Len needed timely explanations and involvement in the discussions. Smith (1998) has commented:

> *'Both the patient's family and caregivers need reassurance that the dementia patient can be kept comfortable without resorting to advanced technological interventions.'*

Control of pain and distress

Ernie suffered from breathlessness (dyspnoea) and from pain induced by handling. There are numerous assessment tools to measure such symptoms. In the main, they are not particularly useful for people with severe dementia. They tend to rely on the understanding of the patient and his or her ability to respond to rating scales. The assessment of pain in dementia is, however, gaining recognition as an issue for research (Cook et al, 1999; Lane et al, 2003).

For the team caring for Ernie, the key to assessment was good observation, a little instinct, and most importantly the experience of knowing him when he was well, relaxed and pain-free. This gave the team a baseline for comparison. The control of symptoms in terminal care will be discussed further in the next chapter.

Rehabilitation and support

In the context of dying, the aim of rehabilitation is to try to ensure that the person's quality of life (including his or her independence) is maintained. This aim is different, however, depending on whether we are discussing palliative care for cognitively intact people with cancer, or for people with severe dementia.

In the case of Ernie, the difficult decisions about hydration and feeding might well be regarded as decisions about the extent to which it was possible to maintain his quality of life. The whole issue of artificial hydration in terminal care is one that brings little consensus among health-care professionals. Opinions can be polarized, but – at least in the field of cancer care – an authoritative body has stated (National Council for Hospice and Specialist Palliative Care Services, 1997):

> *'Towards death, a person's desire for food and drink lessens.*
> *Study evidence is limited... but suggests that artificial hydration in*
> *imminently dying patients influences neither survival nor symptom*
> *control. As such it may constitute an unnecessary intrusion.'*

House (1992) argued that hospital staff appear to allow their own fears to get in the way of what is best for the patient. Nurses polled thought it was unethical and unthinkable not to hydrate. One nurse suggested that artificial hydration benefited the nurse's peace of mind! House (1992) found that junior doctors were more liable to hydrate patients than more senior colleagues, possibly because of lack of experience.

Hospice staff, in comparison, appear to accept the patient's imminent death and do not feel the need to prolong life. House (1992) also said that hospice staff initiated open discussion with carers, offering clear explanations regarding the treatment of symptoms. This reflects the hospice philosophy of care – to give quality to life, not to prolong it. In line with these findings, some of those nursing Ernie were nervous about the lack of hydration, but nevertheless discussed matters openly with Len. Again, these complicated issues will be further discussed later in this book.

However, it is worth noting that just as there are difficult decisions regarding nutrition and hydration, there are similarly problematic decisions in relation to the treatment of infections in severe dementia. In the milder stages of dementia treating infections is not problematic. But later on, the evidence is not so clear; at some stage the treatment would have to be so aggressive that it would become unacceptable, whereas palliative measures might serve the patient just as well (Volicer et al, 1998). In Ernie's case, it had once seemed reasonable to treat his intercurrent infections, but in the terminal phase this no longer seemed appropriate.

Complementary therapies, social and spiritual care

Ernie's social environment required careful attention so that he was not unnecessarily interfered with or distressed by too much activity. In the last days of Ernie's life, however, it was Len's social and spiritual life that required support. In reflecting on these events we are aware that the balance of care sometimes shifted towards Len and away from Ernie. This was not a conscious decision, but was nonetheless important.

Ernie was largely unaware of the quite intensive care he received in his last week of life. The care was delivered with his dignity in mind but because of his condition it was nearly all physical care. Len, on the other hand, was acutely aware of all of the proceedings and was consequently suffering emotional pain. This was recognized by the team and explains why Len became the focus of social support and spiritual concern.

It is also clear, however, that it was Len's standing as the significant relation to Ernie that brought him into the caring context – i.e. the staff's concern for Len was not something in addition to their care for Ernie. It was one and the same thing. And it was a concern that was deeply layered, even to including the dog as an important aspect of care. Similarly, not only touch, but also aromatherapy was used as a means of enhancing the calm environment of care for both Ernie and Len (Thorgrimsen et al, 2003).

The vista that appears when holistic palliative care is taken seriously can be inspiring (Post, 2000):

> *'A new form of hospice for patients with advanced [Alzheimer's disease] would revolve around the concept of "being with" rather than "doing to" patients... Efforts to enhance emotional, relational, and esthetic wellbeing would... involve family members, providing them with a sense of meaning and purpose. Through music, movement therapy, relaxation, and touch, such efforts support patients' remaining capacities. Connections with nature through a beautiful and open environment fit under this rubric, as can spiritual support.'*

Psychological care and bereavement support

People with dementia, even in the severe stages, should receive good quality psychological care. The holistic view means that the psychological needs of the informal carer or relative should also be considered. The hospice approach, sadly lacking in the field of dementia in comparison with cancer care, is likely to pay greater attention to the psychological and physiological needs of dying patients (McArthy et al, 1997).

In our NHS home for people with severe dementia, therefore, part of the purpose of our regular reviews is not only to consider the care of the person with dementia, but also to give the family carers the opportunity to discuss their concerns. As in the case of Len, staff remain very aware of the emotional needs of visiting families and friends.

For many of those close to a person with dementia, once the condition has advanced beyond the milder stages, their experience is that of bereavement – a drawn out, slow form of bereavement. The classical emotional reactions of this in dementia are experienced as in other conditions:

- Shock, numbness, disbelief
- Distress and anger
- Depression and despair
- Acceptance and resolution.

However, these reactions might be passed through at various times (perhaps repeatedly) during the course of an illness that can last, even in its severe forms, for many years. There will still be some sort of bereavement response at the time of death.

Parkes (2000) discusses bereavement in connection with the notion of 'psychosocial transitions'. These are life changes that:

1. Require major revisions of assumptions
2. Are lasting in their implications
3. Take place quickly with little chance for preparation.

It can be seen that dementia fits both of the first two criteria. It could be argued, however, that the changes that occur within dementia might also satisfy the third criterion: the person suddenly becomes violent or disinhibited or incontinent or immobile. He or she may seem to have been in a settled state for many months and then suddenly deteriorates.

Not everyone who is bereaved requires specialist help. Many, like Len, will deal with their bereavements in a natural and individual way. The nature and frequency of contact with the home in which the person with dementia died is often telling. Visiting too frequently for too long may be a sign that the carer cannot 'let go'; but an abrupt cessation of contact after years of almost daily visits may indicate a problem with facing up to the loss.

Many hospices have a form of bereavement service, but for the carers of those who die from dementia the services are little more than embryonic. An inquiring phone call some weeks after the death often depends simply on the informal initiative and concern of a particular nurse or other professional.

The ethics of care

In this chapter we have been considering the holistic view of palliative care and stressing the extent to which this must involve the person's family and friends. Before concluding, it is important to point to the ethical theories that underpin this sort of holism, and highlight two strands of ethical thinking that can be regarded as making up an appropriate ethic of care.

Feminine ethics

Gilligan (1982) argued that, whereas men tend to think of morality in terms of rights, autonomy and justice, for women the key issues are caring, responsibility and inter-relationships. Noddings (1984) suggested a 'feminine' ethic that focused specifically on the idea of caring. Instead of the principles of medical ethics coming as a set of rules, the emphasis was specifically on caring for individuals. This caring is seen as a built-in disposition or virtue, as a constituent part of what it is to be a human being.

The feminine perspective shows the intrinsic importance of our inter-relationships. This has relevance not just for the caring of the nurses for Ernie, but also for Len's caring for Ernie and, therefore, for the nurses' concern for Len.

Inter-relationships are part of what defines us as 'carers'. As professional carers for a person with dementia, we cannot ignore his or her significant relations. They become inevitably involved (even if they choose not to be active) in the nexus of care that surrounds the person.

Narrative ethics

According to narrative ethics, we will only understand the rightness or wrongness of a decision or action if we consider it within the context of the story as a whole (Jones, 1999). We are embedded in our own narratives. But we are never the sole authors of our stories. We interconnect. The story of Ernie inevitably involves Len and vice versa. If we now interact with Ernie as doctors and nurses, inevitably we must interconnect at some level with Len.

Narrative ethics might appear too relativistic to be a moral code, as if almost any story could be acceptable. However, the narratives need to relate and interconnect. While narrative ethics emphasizes interconnectedness and feminine ethics stresses inter-relationships, they share in common an underlying philosophical perspective that sees us as beings who are situated in a shared public space of culture and values (Hughes, 2001). Within this space, the holistic view suggests that the palliative care approach towards people with dementia must inevitably involve concern for those who are significant in their lives.

Conclusion

In caring for people, we ourselves become significant in the lives of all those concerned. As health-care workers, therefore, we must never underestimate the unique role that we have in caring for people with dementia and their families at the time of death. For their relatives and carers the memories of this time will be coloured by our actions, be they for good or ill. Embracing holistic palliative care should help to ensure that the transition from life to death is perhaps made with sadness but without trauma.

References

Cook AK, Niven CA, Downs MG (1999) Assessing the pain of people with cognitive impairment. *Int J Geriatr Psychiatr* **14**(6): 421–5

Department of Health (2001) *National Service Framework for Older People*. Department of Health, London

Gilligan C (1982) *In a Different Voice: Psychological Theory and Women's Development*. Harvard University Press, MA, USA

House N (1992) The hydration question. Hydration or dehydration of terminally ill patients. *Prof Nurse* **8**(1): 44–8

Hughes JC (2001) Views of the person with dementia. *J Med Ethics* **27**(2): 86–91

Jones AH (1999) Narrative based medicine: narrative in medical ethics. *Br Med J* **318**(7178): 253–6

Kitwood T (1997) *Dementia Reconsidered: The Person Comes First*. Open University Press, Buckingham and Philadelphia

Lane P, Kuntupis M, MacDonald S et al (2003) A pain assessment tool for people with advanced Alzheimer's and other progressive dementias. *Home Healthc Nurse* **21**(1): 32–7

McArthy M, Addington-Hall J, Altmann D (1997) The experience of dying with dementia: a retrospective study. *Int J Geriatr Psychiatr* **12**(3): 404–40

National Council for Hospice and Specialist Palliative Care Services (1997) *Ethical Decision-making in Palliative Care: Artificial Hydration for People who are Terminally Ill*. National Council for Hospice and Specialist Palliative Care Services, London

Noddings N (1984) *Caring: A Feminine Approach to Ethics and Moral Education*. University of California Press, Berkeley

Parkes CM (2000) Bereavement as a psychosocial transition. In: Dickenson D, Johnson M, Katz JS (eds) *Death, Dying and Bereavement*. Open University and Sage, London: 325–31

Post SG (2000) *The Moral Challenge of Alzheimer Disease: Ethical Issues from Diagnosis to Dying*. 2nd edn. Johns Hopkins University Press, Baltimore: 107

Smith SJ (1998) Providing palliative care for the terminal Alzheimer patient. In: Volicer L, Hurley A (eds) *Hospice Care for Patients with Advanced Progressive Dementia*. Springer, New York: 247–56

Thorgrimsen L, Spector A, Wiles A, Orrell M (2003) Aromatherapy for dementia. In: *The Cochrane Library*. Issue 4. John Wiley, Chichester

Volicer L, Brandeis GH, Hurley AC (1998) Infections in advanced dementia. In: Volicer L, Hurley A (eds) *Hospice Care for Patients with Advanced Progressive Dementia*. Springer, New York: 29–47

Key points

- The need for palliative care services in severe dementia is often overlooked.

- A holistic view implies that the person with dementia will be cared for in the broadest sense.

- This will, therefore, inevitably involve concern for those close to the person with dementia; they will require physical, psychological, social and spiritual support, along with appropriate help with bereavement.

- The holistic view, bringing in the concerns of others, is supported by the ethics of care, which stresses our interrelationships and interconnectedness.

Chapter 3

Managing the physical symptoms of dying

Claud Regnard, Margaret E Huntley

A fundamental principle in both supportive care and palliative care is to create a 'safe place to suffer' (Stedeford, 1987). At first reading this seems paradoxical since, after all, palliative care is supposed to ease all suffering. But on closer examination the statement can be seen as a logical, pragmatic and sensible underpinning of effective care (*Table 3.1*). The process of expressing suffering will not occur while a patient is in pain, nauseated, breathless or constipated.

Control of physical symptoms is an essential first step if the patient is to feel safe enough to express how he or she feels by whatever means available. Understanding the symptoms requires an understanding of the patient's language of distress and this becomes increasingly important as the patient's breadth of communication narrows.

In this chapter we shall consider some of the commoner symptoms and signs through the eyes of Molly, a (fictional) patient with severe dementia.

Distress

Identifying distress

'I know my name is Molly, but I don't know where I am. I'm in a large room full of people, but I don't know them and they don't speak to me. Sometimes two strangers come along and shout in my ear: "We'll take you to the toilet, love". They attach me to this lifting machine and next thing I'm dangling in the air. I'm scared. I'm frightened – I don't know these people. Why can't I go to the toilet by myself? I'm not silly, you know – they don't understand that. They don't need to shout either, I'm not deaf. I struggle to get out of the machine.

'A woman comes up to me and says, "Hello mum". She's not my daughter – I'm only 30 and she's more than that, but I can't find the words to tell her, and that's frightening. The woman who says she's my

---

Table 3.1: Palliative care: a safe place to suffer

- Effective physical symptom control is the essential first step
- Some psychological suffering will be left – removal of the suffering is not always possible
- However, it is therapeutic for this suffering to be expressed
- Expression will only occur if the patient feels it is safe to do so (and physical symptom control has been effective)
- Expression can be enabled almost anywhere

---

daughter says I'm 86 and a bit confused. She's got the wrong person but she won't go away. It's like a bad dream and I start screaming.'

The language of distress

Despite her communication difficulties, Molly is communicating but she does this differently in a way that has been termed 'alternative communication' (Glennen, 1997). There is a surprising lack of published research on alternative communication in adults like Molly (Tuffrey-Wijne, 2003). Selekman and Malloy (1995) observed that adult carers subconsciously identify 'cues': the recognition of distress by carers seems to be an implicit, rather than explicit, act. The cues consist of a range of fairly obvious signs and behaviours (*Figure 3.1*), but they are neither routinely documented nor monitored. The consequence is that carers are often uncertain about the interpretation of such cues.

The literature has focused on pain, but there is no evidence to support assumptions that signs or behaviours associated with a physical cause, such as pain, are different when compared to the signs or behaviours associated with psychological distress, such as anxiety (Regnard et al, 2003). This is not surprising since pain is a distressing experience. Some patients with Alzheimer's dementia have been observed to have little reaction to painful events, such as fractures (Fisher-Morris and Gellatly, 1997). One hypothesis is that fear, which is a major component of distress, requires some form of memory. So the absence of fear, because of poor memory, will inevitably reduce overall distress. There is no evidence, however, that people with communication difficulties are less sensitive to pain.

Making sense of distress

Pattern recognition of distress signs and behaviours is a crucial step that is missing from much of the work on distress in people with severe communication difficulties.

In palliative care this pattern recognition has been used to produce clinical

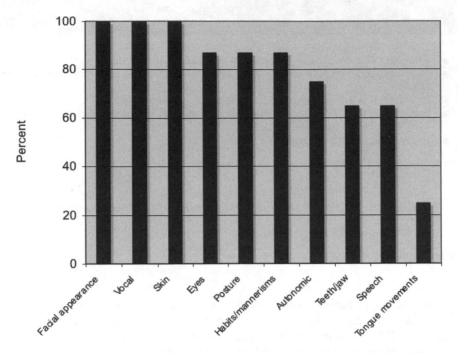

Figure 3.1: Patients with severe communication difficulties showing changes in signs and behaviour during distress (Regnard et al, 2003)

decision flow diagrams and protocols for patients with advanced disease, mainly cancer, who can communicate (Regnard and Hockley, 2003). Several steps in identifying distress can be outlined – these have potential applications in any client who is unable to communicate effectively, including those with dementia (Regnard et al, 2003):

1. A content situation is the one least likely to be associated with distress. It is important to document the signs and behaviour during a content situation if changes are to be noted
2. Any change away from a content behaviour should be documented, especially as distress may be an absence of content signs and behaviours
3   These changes should be checked against the signs and behaviours during previous, known episodes of distress – e.g. constipation or fear of venepuncture
4. The changes observed and the circumstances in which they occurred can then be checked against clinical decision checklists
5. The likeliest cause of the distress is decided, although several possible options may be identified
6. Treatment of the likeliest cause is started
7. The signs and behaviours are rechecked. If they have returned to

baseline (including content signs and behaviour), then the cause and treatment were correct. If there is no change then the second on the treatment list needs to be tried.

Tools to identify distress

Three tools are needed to identify distress.

1. A tool to document the signs and behaviours. Baseline observations need to be documented when the client is content as well as when the client is distressed. The Northgate DisDAT (Disability Distress Assessment Tool) has been developed specifically for this purpose for people with profound communication problems. It differs from previous tools in that it makes no assumptions about the cause of the distress and is not a scoring instrument (Regnard et al, 2003). Such documentation tools enable carers to clarify and record observations they already make.
2. A screening decision checklist (*Table 3.2*). This enables an initial decision to be made on the general cause of the distress.
3. Specific decision checklists for different categories of distress, which have been suggested by the screening checklist, such as fear or pain (Regnard and Hockley, 2003). These are used to narrow down general categories of distress to one, or a few, possible causes which then suggest a specific treatment.

Physical distress

> '*My whole body is sore. It hurts to move and it hurts to sit. A man has come to see me and tells me I have arthritis. I laugh at him and tell him: "At my age? You must be joking!". He tells me I'm 86 and it's common at my age and will give me some medicine. I spit in his face because he's lying.*'

The frequency and severity of physical and psychosocial problems in dementia is very similar to other advanced diseases such as cancer, cardiac disease, respiratory disease, AIDS, and other neurological disease (Addington-Hall et al, 1998). In a small series of people with dementia, 81% had breathlessness, and 59% had pain (Lloyd-Williams, 1996).

A larger series of 170 people with dementia showed that they had needs comparable to cancer patients (McCarthy et al, 1997). In a series of 105 elderly people who could not respond verbally, 78% had pain (Simons and Malabar, 1995).

Table 3.2: Identifying the cause of distress (Regnard and Hockley, 2004)

Is the new sign or behaviour:

Repeated rapidly?
- Consider pleuritic pain (in time with breathing)
- Consider colic (comes and goes every few minutes)
- Consider repetitive movement caused by boredom or fear

Associated with breathing?
- Consider infection, COPD, pleural effusion, cancer

Worsened or precipitated by movement?
- Consider movement-related pains

Related to eating?
- Consider food refusal through illness, fear or depression
- Consider food refusal because of swallowing problems
- Consider upper gastrointestinal problems (oral hygiene, peptic ulcer, dyspepsia) or abdominal problems

Related to a specific situation?
- Consider frightening/painful situations

Associated with vomiting?
- Consider causes of nausea and vomiting

Associated with elimination (urine or faecal)?
- Consider urinary problems (infection, retention)
- Consider gastrointestinal problems (diarrhoea/constipation)

Present in a normally comfortable position or situation?
- Consider pains at rest, infection, nausea

Pain

> *'I don't know how I got here, but I'm in a bed. It hurts when people come and turn me over. They sound so cheerful and I'm unhappy – they keep shouting and I'm not deaf or stupid!'*

Diagnosing the pain

If pain is suspected from the initial distress checklist (*Table 3.2*), it is not acceptable to start an analgesic without making some assessment of the likely cause. This is because the cause of the pain often dictates the treatment and some pains such as colic can be worsened by analgesics such as opioids. Even in severe dementia, where communication is difficult, an assessment of the pain is possible.

Are the signs or behaviours of pain related to movement?
If the slightest movement precipitates the pain then a fracture needs to be excluded by an X-ray. Soft tissue inflammation (e.g. bruising caused by injury or infection) or joint problems (e.g. arthritis) can also cause movement-related pain.

Bone metastases can cause pain when the bone is strained by local pressure or weight-bearing. Skeletal muscle damage or muscle spasm causes pain on active movement. A common muscle pain is myofascial pain caused by the abnormal use of one muscle (e.g. caused by abnormal posture) and it can cause severe pain on movement together with a characteristic tender 'trigger point' in the affected muscle.

Pain synchronized with the movements of breathing suggests a rib problem (e.g. fracture or bone metastasis), pleurisy (e.g. infection, pulmonary embolus, or local cancer) or a chest wall problem (e.g. local tumour). Local rib tenderness on pressure suggests that such a 'breathing pain' is caused by a problem in the rib. Chest pain caused by exercise may suggest angina owing to coronary artery disease.

Are the signs or behaviours of pain periodic?
Pain that repeats regularly every few seconds is likely to be related to breathing. Pain that repeats every few minutes is likely to be colic. This is usually bowel colic (mostly caused by constipation), but it can also be caused by colic of the bladder (e.g. urinary tract infection), uterus (e.g. period pain), gallbladder (e.g. cholecystitis) or ureter (e.g. renal stones or ureteric obstruction by cancer). Bowel colic is the commonest type.

Are the signs and behaviours of pain related to a procedure?
A number of routine procedures can be painful such as taking blood or changing dressings.

Are the signs and behaviours of pain related to eating?
Reduced appetite or food refusal can be caused by pain in the mouth (e.g. dental problems, mucosal infection such as candida, cancer), in the pharynx or oesophagus (e.g. mucosal infection, cancer, acid reflux) or the stomach and duodenum (e.g. gastritis, peptic ulceration or cancer).

Are the signs and behaviours of pain worsened by passing stool or urine?
Urinary causes include urinary tract infections, catheters or the presence of local cancer. Constipation, anal fissures, haemorrhoids and local cancer can cause pain on defaecation.

Are there any associated skin changes in the area of the pain?
Painful skin ulcers can be caused by local pressure damage, skin disease (e.g. dermatitis, psoriasis), local cancer or vascular problems (arterial insufficiency or venous incompetence).

Are the signs or behaviours of pain precipitated by light touch?

Any increased response to touch (hypersensitivity) or pain on touching (allodynia) in a discrete area of skin suggests neuropathic pain. This type of pain is precipitated by nerve damage and can persist long after the cause of the damage has gone. Neuralgia seen after a herpes zoster infection is an example of neuropathic pain, which can persist for years even though the infection heals after a few weeks. Pain in an area of reduced sensation may be caused by nerve compression, such as sciatica.

Are the signs or behaviours of pain persisting?

Unresolved fear, misunderstanding or depression can cause pain to persist. Causes related to medication include analgesics being given too infrequently, doses that are too low, or a preparation that is unpleasant or difficult to take. Finally, persisting pain can be caused by the onset of a new pain. Advice from a pain or palliative care specialist can be helpful when pain persists despite assessment and treatment.

Managing the pain

Even if communication is difficult it is usually possible to narrow down the likely cause of pain to a few choices. Which treatment is used is entirely dependent on the likely cause.

Attempting to treat all pains with the same analgesic will often result in failure or adverse effects. For example, the pain of abdominal colic can be worsened by opioids such as codeine or morphine, while other pains need drugs which are not analgesics but which can relieve pain through indirect mechanisms.

Some pains do not need drug treatment at all. An example is myofascial pain, which can cause troublesome pain on movement and yet is rapidly treated with the application of a transcutaneous electrical nerve stimulator (TENS) or acupuncture. *Table 3.3* shows a summary of first-line treatments for different pains.

Primary and secondary analgesics

Primary analgesics have a direct action on blocking pain pathways. They include non-opioids (e.g. paracetamol), weak opioids (e.g. codeine) and strong opioids (e.g. morphine).

It is usual to start with paracetamol, move to codeine if this is ineffective, and then move to morphine if the pain persists. Secondary analgesics (also called co-analgesics or adjuvant analgesics) relieve pain through an indirect mechanism and include drugs such as hyoscine butylbromide for colic, amitriptyline for neuropathic pain and dexamethasone for nerve compression pain caused by tumour.

It is common to prescribe primary and secondary analgesics together. When the pain is frequent or continuous the analgesic should be prescribed regularly, since using them on an 'as required' basis results in poor pain relief – continuous pain needs continuous analgesia.

Strong opioids
Strong opioids, such as morphine, are effective analgesics that are safe when used correctly. Most are equally effective (i.e. they treat the same range of pains), but some strong opioids are more potent than others (i.e. less of the drug is needed to have the same effect). This does not make them more effective. For example, fentanyl is nearly 150 times more potent than morphine but treats the same range of pains, whereas in contrast, methadone is similar in potency to morphine but can be more effective for some pains such as neuropathic pain.

All opioids are deactivated in the liver with the exception of morphine, which is converted to potent, active metabolites that are excreted through the kidney. Consequently liver disease has only a modest effect on the patient's ability to handle morphine, but any change in kidney function causes the active metabolites to accumulate.

Most other strong opioids are affected by liver disease, but much less affected by kidney disease. There is no standard dose of opioid since the final required dose of a strong opioid cannot be predicted by assessing weight, age, sex or surface area. Consequently, patients already on a full dose of a weak opioid (e.g. 30mg codeine 4-hourly) are started on low doses of a strong opioid (e.g. 20mg controlled-release oral morphine 12-hourly).

Patients are also started on an instant release strong opioid to take for breakthrough pain while the controlled-release dose is being titrated. The dose is then gradually increased (usually in 25–50% steps every 2–3 days) until the patient is comfortable. The median daily dose of oral morphine in cancer care is 100mg, but very few patients need more than 500mg daily.

Adverse effects of analgesics
Paracetamol is usually safe as long as doses are not higher than 1g 4-hourly. In contrast, non-steroidal anti-inflammatory (NSAID) drugs can cause gastric irritation and severe bleeding from the gut and renal damage especially if the patient is dehydrated.

Addiction is not seen in patients taking strong opioids for pain relief (Berger et al, 1998; Borghjerg et al, 1996), their analgesic effect does not wear off, and drug doses do not have to be repeatedly escalated (Taub, 1982).

Strong opioids do not hasten death or shorten life (Regnard and Badger, 1987; Cools et al, 1996; Twycross et al, 2002). Adverse effects are not a problem for most patients as tolerance develops to most adverse effects. Mild drowsiness wears off within a few days, while tolerance to respiratory depression is so rapid that it is rare in the routine use of strong opioids. In contrast, constipation does not wear off and nearly all patients on weak or strong opioids should be

Table 3.3: Methods of treating pain (Regnard and Hockley, 2004)

Pain	First line management
Bone pain owing to metastases or osteoporosis	
Pain on weight bearing or straining the affected bone	Find positions and activities that are least painful Refer to pain or palliative care teams for advice on strong opioids and the use of bisphosphonates. Radiotherapy can reduce pain in 65% of patients with bone metastases
Colic	
Regular pain occurring every few minutes	Treat the cause, e.g; abdominal colic – treat constipation; urinary colic – exclude urinary tract infection or renal stones. If persistent (eg. bowel obstruction owing to cancer) refer to palliative care team for advice on the use of hyoscine butylbromide
Eating-related pain	
Food refusal, pain during eating, swallowing, abdominal pain	Exclude dental problems or oral infection or (candida, herpes simplex or zoster) and refer for treatment. Refer for medical opinion for assessing oesophageal and gastric causes. An antacid may help as a temporary measure
Elimination-related pain	
Pain on passing urine or stool without colic	Constipation: adjust laxatives to produce a comfortable stool. Urinary tract infection: culture urine and treat. Haemorrhoids: use local cream. Local cancer: refer to palliative care team for advice
Exercise chest pain	
Tightness or heaviness in chest, perhaps with breathlessness	Refer for medical opinion to exclude angina
Fracture	
Pain on the slightest passive movement	Refer for X-ray and assessment
Joint pain	
Pain on moving joint, sometimes with local swelling	Refer for medical opinion to assess cause. Paracetamol 1g 4–6 hourly may help, but NSAIDs may be needed
Persisting pain	
Pain persisting despite treatment	Exclude anxiety, anger or depression. Refer to pain or palliative care team for advice

Myofascial pain	
Pain on using affected muscle with local tenderness in the muscle	Local cooling may help. Ask for advice on the use of a TENS, otherwise refer to pain or palliative care team for assessment
Neuropathic pain	
Sensitivity or pain on light touch	Refer to pain or palliative care team for advice on the use of amitriptyline or gabapentin
Procedure pain	
Pain owing to a specific procedure	Modify procedure – e.g. use local anaesthetic cream before taking a blood sample
Skin inflammation	
Redness, ulceration or weeping of skin	Refer for medical opinion to assess cause. Pressure ulcer: institute local pressure care and pressure ulcer policy. Malignant ulcer: refer to palliative care team for advice
Soft tissue injury	
Visible bruising, local pain on pressure	Exclude serious injury. Local cooling may help. If still painful try paracetamol 1g 4–6 hourly

prescribed a laxative. If adverse effects are a problem, there are now effective alternative strong opioids that can be used, such as hydromorphone, oxycodone and fentanyl.

Constipation, nausea and vomiting

'I can get out of bed now. I want to go home, but it hurts when I go to the toilet and I've been sick. People keep giving me food but I don't want to eat – I was sick over one person who kept pushing food into my mouth.'

Constipation

In advanced disease it is common to eat less, and a reduced frequency of bowel motions is normal. Consequently, frequency of passing stool cannot be used as a definition of constipation, whereas a hard stool that is uncomfortable to pass is a more useful indicator.

There are many causes of constipation, including reduced intake of fibre,

Table 3.4: Clinical decisions for managing constipation (Regnard and Hockley, 2004)	
Is this bowel obstruction?	• Refer for a surgical opinion
Is there a treatable cause?	• Correct dehydration or change to less constipating drugs
Is the environment making the person upset?	• Ensure privacy and calm
Is this mild constipation?	• Use a gentle laxative, e.g. docusate
Is the rectum or stoma full?	• Start stimulant and softening laxatives, e.g. senna and docusate
Is the constipation persisting?	• Exclude local rectal problems, e.g. haemorrhoids. Consider using Movicol

reduced fluid intake, drugs that slow the bowel (e.g. analgesics), any cause of dehydration and anything that makes passing stool painful (e.g. local tumour or haemorrhoids).

Table 3.4 outlines the management of constipation. A bowel obstruction needs to be excluded if no stool has been passed at all for more than 5 days. The correct choice of laxative is important. If the constipation is mild, a gentle laxative (e.g. docusate) can help. Lactulose can help in low doses, such as 5–10ml 12-hourly, but higher doses commonly cause abdominal bloating and discomfort.

More troublesome constipation often needs a combination of a stimulant laxative (e.g. senna or bisacodyl) and a softening laxative (e.g. docusate or low-dose lactulose). Danthron is a stimulant laxative that is available in combinations (e.g. co-danthrusate, co-danthramer), but these commercial combinations tend to be expensive. In addition, they can colour the urine red (giving the impression of bleeding) and cause chemical burns around the anus.

If a hard stool is present in the large bowel, Movicol (whose main constituent is macrogol or polyethylene glycol) is a laxative that can help to soften and clear impacted stool, but one sachet must be mixed with exactly 125ml of water to be effective. Impacted stool in the rectum may clear with a suppository, but occasionally a manual evacuation is needed. This is best done under mild sedation for the sake of comfort and kindness.

Nausea and vomiting

Immediate measures for vomiting include a large bowl, tissues and water to rinse out the mouth. When vomiting is the main problem with little or no nausea, the reason may be gastric stasis caused by poor gastric emptying, which responds to drugs that encourage normal gastric emptying (e.g. domperidone or metoclopramide). Rarer causes of vomiting with little or no nausea include oesophageal obstruction or raised intracranial pressure.

There are many causes of nausea. Chemical causes (drugs, hypercalcaemia, bacterial toxins) will often respond to low doses of haloperidol (0.5–1.5mg once at night). An ear infection needs to be excluded if the nausea or vomiting is related to movement. Other reasons for nausea or vomiting include gastric irritation (caused by non-steroidal anti-inflammatory drugs – NSAIDs – or steroids, for example) and the effects of fear or anxiety.

Nausea or vomiting that persists may respond to cyclizine or levomepromazine. Many antiemetics (drugs that prevent vomiting) need to be given by parenteral routes initially and metoclopramide, haloperidol and levomepromazine can all be given subcutaneously. Domperidone can be given rectally.

Breathing problems

> *'My breathing is getting worse and it's too hot in here. When I cough someone sticks a tube down my throat. I just need to open a window – that would help my breathing.'*

Breathlessness can be common and the sensation can be eased by simple measures that can be started by any carer (*Table 3.5*). Sudden or severe breathlessness requires an urgent assessment and may need specialist advice since some causes can be treated and reversed (Regnard and Hockley, 2003).

Assessment and treatment are often worthwhile. For example, it is common for older patients who are ill to be nursed flat, which can precipitate an episode of distressing breathlessness caused by ventricular failure. This is rapidly

Table 3.5: Simple measures for breathlessness

- Call for help
- Sit the patient upright
- Increase air movement over the patient's face (use a gentle fan or open a window)
- Help the patient relax the shoulders by massaging them in a downwards direction (this reverses the 'hunching' caused by anxiety and increases the capacity to breathe)
- Explain what is happening and stay with the patient

Table 3.6: Goals in the care pathway for the dying patient (Ellershaw and Ward, 2003)

- Current medication is assessed and non-essentials discontinued:
  Stop all non-essential medication and if unable to swallow convert to
  sub-cutaneous (SC) route or once-daily preparations
- As required subcutaneous medication written up as follows:

Pain:	If not on oral morphine use or prescribe diamorphine 2.5mg SC 4-hourly if required (PRN)
	If already on morphine, convert to a diamorphine SC infusion (ask palliative care team for advice on conversions)
Nausea and vomiting:	Use or prescribe cyclizine 25–50mg SC 8-hourly PRN
Respiratory tract secretions:	Use or prescribe hyoscine hydrobromide 400mg SC 8-hourly PRN
Terminal restlessness and agitation:	Continue previous analgesic requirements but avoid using opioids to sedate since there is a risk of increasing the agitation
	Use or prescribe midazolam 5–10mg SC 1–2 hourly PRN

- Discontinue inappropriate interventions (e.g. regular blood test)
- Assess the ability to communicate in English
- Assess the patient's insight into his or her condition
- Assess his or her religious and spiritual needs
- Identify how the family and others are to be informed of the patient's impending death
- Give family and other relevant people the information they need
- Ensure that all the key people are aware of the patient's condition
- Discuss and explain the plan of care with the patient (if possible) and the family
- Ensure that the family and other people involved understand the plan of care

reversed by intravenous or intramuscular furosemide and by ensuring that the patient is nursed sitting or semi-prone.

With regard to chest infections, staff can be concerned as to whether treatment is ethically justified when this could prolong a patient's distress. In the context of dementia it has been argued that withholding antibiotics, but providing palliative measures (e.g. antipyretics and analgesia), neither accelerates the progression of the disease nor increases distress (Volicer et al, 1998). However, clinical experience elsewhere suggests that treating a chest infection with an antibiotic is the simplest and quickest way to relieve distress.

In palliative care more generally, even in the terminal stages there is evidence that the use of antibiotics is helpful in relieving the distress of infected bronchial secretions (Spruyt and Kausae, 1998; Clayton et al, 2003). When bronchial secretions are not caused by infection or ventricular failure, but are related to the terminal nature of the illness, hyoscine hydrobromide can be used (*Table 3.6*).

When fear accompanies the breathlessness this can be helped by applying the simple measures outlined in *Table 3.5*, but occasionally the fear is severe and may need medication. Opioids can help breathlessness and are safe when they are titrated in the same way as for pain (Boyd and Kelly, 1997; Flowers, 2003). However, opioids make poor sedatives since rapid titration can cause adverse effects, which include increased agitation, while tolerance to drowsiness develops within days. Lorazepam 0.5–1mg orally provides relaxation with minimal sedation. Breathlessness that is more severe and persistent needs the advice of a palliative care specialist.

Problems with nutrition and hydration

> *'I'm thirsty, but don't want to drink. Every time I try to drink I just end up coughing. Food is worse – some gets stuck and that's very frightening.'*

Where there are problems with feeding and drinking, a range of questions needs to be considered:

Is the prognosis short?

When the prognosis is very short (i.e. hour-by-hour or day-by-day deterioration) then hydration and nutrition are solely for comfort and pleasure. Most patients only need sips of water for comfort and it is rare for a patient to feel hungry. Comatose and comfortable patients need only good mouth care to keep the mouth moist.

Is there a request to withdraw hydration or feeding?

When a competent patient who is not depressed refuses hydration or feeding with the full understanding that this may shorten his or her life, the patient's choice needs to be respected. Patients with advanced dementia are unlikely

> **Table 3.7: Hints for determining best interests (Lord Chancellor's Department, 2003)**
>
> - Find out the past and present wishes and feelings of the person and the factors which the person would consider if he or she were able to do so
> - Allow and encourage the person to participate, or improve his or her ability to participate, as fully as possible in the decision-making process
> - Consult relatives and others, where appropriate and practical, about the person's wishes and feelings and what would be in his or her best interests
> - Explore any other possible options or alternatives available for achieving the proposed outcome, and consider which option would allow most freedom for the person's future

to be competent in the required sense. In this situation the clinical team has to make a decision on their behalf and in their best interests, where these are understood broadly (*Table 3.7*).

There will be several issues for staff and family to take into account as they consider the patient's best interests:

- The reality of stopping hydration and feeding: although the dying phase in most patients lasts only a few days, a fasting individual can survive for more than 60 days without feeding (Cranford, 1991). In addition, the process of protein, fat and carbohydrate breakdown produces water so that humans can survive for long periods with surprisingly small amounts of water. A possible result of stopping hydration and feeding is that patients do not die, but live to develop nutritional deficiency problems such as pressure ulcers.
- The pitfalls associated with estimating the patient's quality of life: there is good evidence that estimates of a patient's quality of life by health professionals often do not match the patient's own view (Donnelly, 2001; Mencap, 2001). Clinical decisions should be based on whether an intervention is realistic, practical or beneficial.
- The risks of using food refusal as an indicator of a competent choice: there are many reasons for food refusal that have nothing to do with a competent desire to stop eating or drinking. For example, nasogastric tubes are widely disliked by patients and attempting to pull one out only confirms this dislike while revealing nothing about the patient's wishes concerning hydration or feeding.

When the prognosis is longer (i.e. week-by-week deterioration or slower), nutrition and hydration are important to maintain comfort and avoid the problems of nutritional deficiency such as pressure ulcers.

Hence, this rarely presents as an ethical dilemma, but rather as a clinical issue to do with maintaining comfort. The reality is that stopping nutrition and hydration too soon does not result in a rapid deterioration but in prolonged discomfort.

Is the patient anxious or withdrawn?

Depression or anxiety are potent causes of a refusal to eat or drink and in many patients the two co-exist. Treating depression is often worthwhile and will reduce co-existing anxiety, while managing anxiety alone will reduce a patient's distress.

Are swallowing problems present?

Dysphagia is a common problem in dementia (Wasson et al, 2001). Localization by the patient is often accurate while food consistencies are unreliable indicators and the gag reflex is of little value in assessing the cause.

Having excluded oral problems (dental problems, candida, local tumour), further assessment is important. If the food sticks at the level of the chest or abdomen then referral to a gastroenterologist is necessary. However, if the problem is felt to be at the level of the mouth or pharynx, an assessment by a swallowing therapist is important. (Chapter 10 considers swallowing problems.)

If swallowing is sufficiently compromised to reduce intake and the cause is not treatable, then non-oral feeding should be considered. Short-term non-oral hydration can be managed with subcutaneous hydration, which is now a well-established technique (Fainsinger et al, 1994).

Nasogastric tubes are poorly tolerated by patients, do not increase survival and may worsen aspiration (Scott and Austin, 1994; Finucane and Bynum, 1996; Mitchell et al, 1997). Gastrostomies are a better-tolerated alternative (Hull et al, 1993). One study suggested they were less well tolerated in patients with dementia (Sanders et al, 2000), but the experience of one of us (Claud Regnard) in Down's-related dementia is that gastrostomies are well tolerated for long periods.

Are physical symptoms present?

Many physical problems can cause reduced appetite or food refusal. These include oral problems, pain, nausea, vomiting, constipation, dyspepsia, fatigue and disability. Other possibilities are altered taste caused by zinc deficiency, vitamin B deficiency, drugs (eg. phenytoin, flurazepam), dry mouth or concurrent systemic disease.

Is the feeding tube blocked?

Flushing a blocked gastrostomy tube with 30ml of warm water may help; followed, if necessary, by 30ml of carbonated water. If the tube is still blocked, inserting 30ml of pineapple juice may help if left for one hour before flushing. It is also important to avoid giving antacids, diazepam and phenytoin with feeds since these may block tubes. Some preparations, such as crushed enteric-coated tablets or capsule contents, may also cause blockages.

Could drugs be the cause?

Consider drugs that cause nausea (e.g. opioids, metronidazole, trimethoprim), mucosal irritation (e.g. NSAIDs, chemotherapy, antibiotics), delayed gastric emptying (e.g. opioids, amitriptyline, cyclizine) or drugs with central appetite suppressant effects (e.g. opioids, amphetamines).

Is the food presentation or environment a problem?

Poor food presentation, unpleasant odours, a lack of privacy and a lack of help can all reduce intake.

Confusional states

> *They are watching me from the door, waiting to hurt me. I can hear them talking about me, plotting a moment to catch me out. I am so frightened, but they keep me locked up here.*

Differentiating an acute confusional state from the chronic confusional state of dementia can be difficult. Unlike a chronic confusional state, the onset of an acute confusional state is rapid (hours or days), the confusion fluctuates during the day and alertness is altered (increased or decreased). In addition, disorganized thinking, memory impairment, psychomotor activity

Table 3.8: Clinical decision for an acute confusional state

Is memory impairment worse than usual?	• Increase the number, availability and frequency of orientation in time, place and person
Has alertness changed?	• Consider these causes: drugs (started or stopped), recent trauma or infection, biochemical, hormonal, or cardiac problems
Is concentration impaired?	• eg. pain, breathlessness, anxiety, depression.
Is urgent control of disturbance necessary?	• Ensure a light, quiet environment with a minimum of staff changes
	• In the absence of abnormal experiences or behaviour: benzodiazepine (eg. lorazepam)
	• In the presence of abnormal experiences or behaviour: antipsychotic (eg. haloperidol)

and inattention may all worsen (O'Keefe and Lavan, 1999). In the presence of dementia it is important to think of an acute confusional state (or delirium) before assuming that the symptoms are a behavioural problem of dementia, because acute confusional states can often be treated.

The decisions involved in assessing and treating an acute confusional state are summarized in *Table 3.8*.

Is memory impairment worse than usual?

In dementia there is a failure to retain information, but an acute confusional state also causes a failure to take in information, making memory failure seem worse. The patient can be re-orientated by increasing the number, availability and frequency of 'reality clues' about time, place and person.

Has alertness changed?

This supports the presence of an acute confusional state. Possibilities are drugs that have been recently started or stopped, remembering that the long half lives of some drugs mean that it may take days or weeks for the effects to appear. Other common causes are infection, biochemical causes (e.g. dehydration, uraemia, hypercalcaemia, inappropriate antidiuretic hormone secretion), hormonal causes (e.g. thyroid, pituitary or adrenal abnormalities), cardiac problems (e.g. ventricular failure, arrhythmias), hypoxia (e.g. pulmonary metastases, embolism, pleural effusion), or recent trauma (long bone fracture, subdural haematoma). Treatment will depend on the cause.

Is concentration impaired?

If anxiety is present, this may be distracting the patient from taking in information. Calm reassurance can help, but some patients may be too frightened to pay attention and may need help with medication (see below). In the absence of anxiety, other causes of distraction need to be excluded such as a physical symptom (e.g. pain) or a psychiatric illness (e.g. depression).

Is urgent control of disturbance necessary?

Drugs should be a last resort (Drug and Therapeutics Bulletin, 2003). Ensuring a light, quiet environment with a minimum of staff changes and calm re-orientation can help. (For a discussion of the importance of the environment in these circumstances, see Chapter 7.) Occasionally, however, the behaviour risks harm to the confused patient or others, or there is a clear consensus that the patient is very distressed by the experience. Drugs should be chosen on the basis of the symptoms (Conn and Lief, 2001). In the absence of abnormal behaviour, and in the presence of anxiety, benzodiazepines will help suppress the anxiety to a level that is manageable for the patient. However, benzodiazepines can worsen confusion (Breitbart et al, 1996), and when abnormal behaviour or severe anxiety is present then antipsychotic medication is needed. A few patients need both. It is unusual to need to sedate a confused patient (Conn and Lief, 2001), but irreversible confusion causing persistent suffering in the last hours and days of a patient's life may need drugs and doses that cause sedation (Cheng et al, 2001; Chiu, 2001; Fainsinger, 2000; Fainsinger, 1998).

The last hours and days

'I look around and I'm all alone. Where am I? Where is my husband, Wilf?
He should be with me. I drift to sleep and wake to see a woman in the chair
beside me. I look and see her face – it's my daughter, but doesn't she look
older! I tell her I love her and ask for Wilf. "He's dead" she says.

I cry before drifting off to sleep. I wake to find someone pushing something in my mouth. They tell me kindly they're just cleaning my mouth. They hold my hand and give me a kiss on the forehead before leaving. I see my daughter and recognize that I'm an old woman now, my husband is dead and she is grieving for me even though I'm still here. I'm so tired and drained.'

Some carers find it difficult to diagnose the onset of dying, but there are signs and behaviours that suggest a patient has entered the last hours and days (*Table 3.9*). If the team is clear that this is the situation then a number of goals in the care pathway for the dying patient (CPDP) need to be achieved (*Table 3.6*) (Ellershaw and Ward, 2003). Following these goals will help most patients, but if the treatments are unhelpful or cannot be used it is important to contact the local palliative care team for advice. Many hospices provide 24-hour telephone advice.

Persisting agitation in the last hours and days is unusual, but it is distressing to all when it occurs and it is important to reduce the distress. Other than continuing previous analgesic requirements, opioids should not be used for sedation as they risk increasing the agitation. In contrast, low doses of subcutaneous midazolam can be helpful and can be given by a continuous subcutaneous infusion. Other drugs are occasionally needed and a palliative care team can advise which would be most appropriate.

Since the patient is dying naturally of his or her disease, resuscitation would be of no benefit to the patient. Consequently there is no resuscitation decision to be made, only a 'Do Not Attempt Resuscitation' order to be documented. This means that relatives do not have to be asked for permission not to resuscitate, but they must be kept informed of this fact and of any developments as in the five final goals of the CPDP (*Table 3.6*).

In most cases, following the CPDP will allow a patient to die comfortably and peacefully. In many cases it is more a gentle winding down than any sudden presence of death and it is the partner, family, staff and friends who need most of the care and support.

More information is available on palliative care generally (Doyle et al, 2003), on symptom control (Regnard and Hockley, 2004) and on pharmacological aspects of palliative care (Twycross et al, 2002). Foundation texts (Regnard and Kindlen, 2002) and learning materials (Regnard, 2004) are also available.

Table 3.9: Signs and behaviours that suggest a patient with dementia is dying (Regnard and Hockley, 2003)

- Deteriorating day-by-day or faster
- Increasingly drowsy or comatose
- Increasingly bed-bound
- Peripherally cyanosed and cold
- Taking increasingly little food, fluid or oral medication
- Altered breathing pattern

References

Addington-Hall J, Fakhoury W, McCarthy M (1998) Specialist palliative care in non-malignant disease. *Palliat Med* **12**: 417–27

Berger AM, Portenoy R, Weissman DE (1998) Substance abuse issues in palliative care. In: Berger AM (ed) *Principles and Practice of Supportive Oncology.* Lippincott-Raven, Philadelphia

Borgbjerg FM, Nielsen K, Franks J (1996) Experimental pain stimulates respiration and attenuates morphine-induced respiratory depression: a controlled study in human volunteers. *Pain* **64**(1): 123–8

Boyd KJ, Kelly M (1997) Oral morphine as symptomatic treatment of dyspnoea in patients with advanced cancer. *Palliat Med* **11**(4): 277–81

Breitbart W, Marotta R, Platt MM et al (1996) A double-blind trial of haloperidol, chlorpromazine, and lorazepam in the treatment of delirium in hospitalized AIDS patients. *Am J Psychiatry* **153**(2): 231-7

Cheng C, Roemer-Becuwe C, Pereira J (2002) Clinical note. When midazolam fails. *J Pain Symptom Manage* **23**(3): 256-65

Chiu T, Hu W, Lue B, Cheng S, Chen C (2001) Sedation for refractory symptoms of terminal cancer patients in Taiwan. *J Pain Symptom Manage* **21**(6): 467-72

Clayton J, Fardell B, Hutton-Potts J et al (2003) Parenteral antibiotics in a palliative care unit: prospective analysis of current practice. *Palliat Med* **17**(1): 44–8

Cools HJ, Berkhout AM, De Bock GH (1996) Subcutaneous morphine infusion by syringe driver for terminally ill patients. *Age Ageing* **25**(3): 206–8

Conn DK, Lieff S (2001) Diagnosing and managing delirium in the elderly. *Can Fam Physician* **47**(January): 101-8

Cranford RE (1991) Neurologic syndromes and prolonged survival: when can artificial nutrition and hydration be forgone? *Law Med Health Care* **19**(1–2): 13–22

Donnelly M (2001) Decision-making for mentally incompetent people: the empty formula of best interests? *Med Law* **20**(3): 405–16

Doyle D, Hanks G, Cherney NI, Calman K (eds) (2004) *Oxford Textbook of Palliative Medicine.* 3rd edn. Oxford University Press, Oxford

Drug and Therapeutics Bulletin (2003) Drugs for disruptive features in dementia. *Drug Ther Bull* **41**(1): 1-4

Ellershaw J, Ward C (2003) Care of the dying patient: the last hours or days of life. *Br Med J* **326**(7379): 30–4

Fainsinger RL, MacEachern T, Miller MJ et al (1994) The use of hypodermoclysis for rehydration in terminally ill cancer patients. *J Pain Symptom Manage* **9**(5): 298–302

Fainsinger RL, Landman W, Hoskings M, Bruera E (1998) Sedation for uncontrolled symptoms in a South African hospice. *J Pain Symptom Manage* **16**(3): 145-52

Fainsinger RL, Waller A, Bercovici M et al (2000) A multicentre international study of sedation for uncontrolled symptoms in terminally ill patients. *Palliat Med* **14**(4): 257-65

Finucane TE, Bynum JP (1996) Use of tube feeding to prevent aspiration pneumonia. *Lancet* **348**(9039): 1421–4

Fisher-Morris M, Gellatly A (1997) The experience and expression of pain in Alzheimer patients. *Age Ageing 26*(6): 497–500

Flowers B (2003) Palliative care for patients with end-stage heart failure. *Nurs Times* **99**(11): 30–2

Glennen SL (1997) Introduction to augmentative and alternative communication. In: Glennen ST, DeCoste DC (eds) *Handbook of Augmentative and Alternative Communication*. Singular Publishing Group, San Diego: 3–19

Hull MA, Rawlings J, Murray J et al (1993) Audit of outcome of long-term enteral nutrition by percutaneous endoscopic gastrostomy. *Lancet* **341**(8849): 869–72

Lloyd-Williams M (1996) An audit of palliative care in dementia. *Eur J Cancer Care* **5**(1): 53–5

Lord Chancellor's Department (2003) *Making Decisions: A Guide for Healthcare Professionals*. Lord Chancellor's Department, London

McCarthy M, Addington-Hall J, Altmann D (1997) The experience of dying with dementia: a retrospective study. *Int J Geriatr Psychiatr* **12**(3): 404–9

Mencap (2001) *'Quality of life' and medical decision making for adults with profound and multiple learning disabilities*. www.mencap.org.uk/html/campaigns/health_pubs.htm (accessed 24 February 2004)

Mitchell SL, Kiely DK, Lipsitz LA (1997) The risk factors and impact on survival of feeding tube placement in nursing home residents with severe cognitive impairment. *Arch Intern Med* **157**(3): 327–32

O'Keeffe ST, Lavan JN (1999) Clinical significance of delirium subtypes in older people. *Age Ageing* **28**(2): 115-9

Regnard C (ed) (2004) *Helping the Patient with Advanced Disease: A Workbook*. Radcliffe Medical Press, Oxford

Regnard C, Badger C (1987) Opioids, sleep and the time of death. *Palliat Med* **1**(2): 107–10

Regnard C, Hockley J (2003) *A Guide to Symptom Relief in Palliative Care*. 5th edn. Radcliffe Medical Press, Oxford

Regnard C, Kindlen M (2002) *Supportive and Palliative Care in Cancer: An Introduction*. Radcliffe Medical Press, Oxford

Regnard C, Matthews D, Gibson L et al (2003) Difficulties in identifying distress and its causes in people with severe communication problems. *Int J Palliat Nurs* **9**(4): 173–6

Sanders DS, Carter MJ, D'Silva J et al (2000) Survival analysis in percutaneous endoscopic gastrostomy feeding: a worse outcome in patients with dementia. *Am J Gastroenterol* **95**(6): 1472–5

Scott AG, Austin HE (1994) Nasogastric feeding in the management of severe dysphagia in motor neurone disease. *Palliat Med* **8**(1): 45–9

Selekman J, Malloy E (1995) Difficulties in symptom recognition in infants. *J Paediatr Nurs* **10**(2): 89–92

Simons W, Malabar R (1995) Assessing pain in elderly patients who cannot respond verbally. *J Adv Nurs* **22**(4): 663–9

Spruyt O, Kausae A (1998) Antibiotic use for infective terminal respiratory secretions. *J Pain Symptom Manage* **15**(5): 263–4

Stedeford A (1987) A safe place to suffer. *Palliat Med* **1**: 73–4

Taub A (1982) Opioid analgesics in the treatment of chronic intractable pain of non-neoplastic origin. In: Kitahata LM, Collins JG (eds) *Narcotic Analgesics in Anaesthesiology*. Williams and Wilkins, Baltimore: 199–208

Tuffrey-Wijne I (2003) The palliative care needs of people with intellectual disabilities: a literature review. *Palliat Med* **17**(1): 55–62

Twycross RG, Wilcock A, Charlesworth S (eds) (2002) *Palliative Care Formulary*. 2nd edn. (PCF-2). Radcliffe Medical Press, Oxford. www.palliativedrugs.com (accessed 23 January 2004)

Volicer L, Brandeis GH, Hurley AC (1998) Infections in advanced dementia. In: Volicer L, Hurley A (eds) *Hospice Care for Patients with Advanced Progressive Dementia*. Springer, New York: 29–47

Wasson K, Tate H, Hayes C (2001) Food refusal and dysphagia in older people with dementia: ethical and practical issues. *Int J Palliat Nurs* **7**(10): 465–71

Key points

- Suffering can only be expressed in a safe place, where physical symptoms are controlled.

- This requires an understanding of the language of distress.

- Careful observation of when a person is content, and when not, will allow carers to pick up the signs and behaviours of distress.

- Pain can be assessed, even in severe dementia, and rational treatments planned.

- Different pains must be treated differently.

- Specialist palliative care teams are always willing to advise on symptom management.

- Recognising the approach of death allows carers to take steps that are appropriate to the dying phase of the illness, in keeping with the goals of the care pathway for the dying patient (CPDP).

- Dealing with the ethical issues that arise in connection with terminal care requires a clear understanding of the relevant facts.

Chapter 4

The ethics of end-of-life decisions in severe dementia

Julian C Hughes, Philip Dove

What are the ethical issues that arise in nursing homes for people with severe dementia at the end of their lives? The short answer is that they are many and various, because all clinical decisions give rise to ethical concerns at some level. No treatment decision, or decision not to treat, is ethically neutral. Such decisions always involve values as well as facts.

In this chapter we shall consider: the principles of medical ethics and advance directives; the notion of futility in connection with resuscitation; the distinction between ordinary and extraordinary means as they relate to treatment decisions; the principle of double effect and the distinction between acts and omissions in connection with a discussion of euthanasia. We shall end by advocating a perspective that stresses the virtues. The question then is: what do we become by doing or not doing whatever it is? The answer to this question should guide our treatment decisions. In this chapter we focus on the professional perspective. In Chapter 9 Clive Baldwin discusses the family carers' perspectives on ethical issues.

Principles and advance directives

Nowadays many health care workers will have heard of the four principles of medical ethics:

1. Beneficence – doing good
2. Non-maleficence – avoiding harm
3. Autonomy – respecting the person's right to make decisions
4. Justice – acting fairly (Beauchamp and Childress, 2001).

These principles would certainly be useful in thinking about problems at the end of life. Relieving the person's suffering and minimizing the chances of harm (i.e. beneficence and non-maleficence) are clearly important at the end of life. In addition, the issue of fairness (i.e. justice) would have to be taken into account: by treating this person with extra nursing, do I detract from the care of other needy patients?

The principle that has come to dominate, however, is the principle of autonomy. This stresses that we must respect the person's own decisions. The problem in severe dementia is that we may not know the person's real views. One solution is the advance directive or 'living will'. On a properly drawn up and witnessed document, people can state what they would want to happen to them if they were to become 'incompetent'. There are, however, a number of problems with advance directives. In particular, it is difficult to know, some years on perhaps, whether the circumstances that now obtain were the ones the person anticipated when they said (for example) that they would not wish to have antibiotics if they had dementia.

The advance directive has to be seen in the light of concrete circumstances (Hughes and Louw, 2005). In this light it may be a useful tool in deciding what is best for the person; but it is not the only tool. The person's currently expressed views (if known), the views of the relevant friends and family, the views of the carers and the rest of the multidisciplinary team, should all be taken into account, along with the general need to do good and avoid harm.

Perhaps the clearest statement of this thought is to be found in the UK Government's discussion paper *Who Decides?* (Lord Chancellor's Department, 1997):

> *'The advanced statement is not...to be seen in isolation, but against a background of doctor/patient dialogue and the involvement of other carers who may be able to give an insight as to what the patient would want in the particular circumstances of the case.'*

The interesting point is that the way in which advance directives cannot be taken in isolation mirrors the way in which thinkers have gradually allowed that autonomy has to be regarded more broadly too. 'Actual autonomy' is a matter of 'everyday actions in the shared world of social life' (Agich, 2003). Autonomy has to be understood in the context of our interdependency.

In severe dementia, therefore, decisions about end-of-life matters will require attention to broader principles: not just a respect for the person's autonomy, but a respect for that autonomy in the midst of competing concerns. Vallis and Boyd (2002) identified three further relevant principles in end-of-life decisions:

1. *Protective responsibility:* where the professional has a responsibility to protect vulnerable patients from harm
2. *Responsibility for narrative integrity:* which involves knowing people well and defending their best interests
3. *Candour:* where this means being completely open and truthful.

These further principles bring in the idea of 'relationship' and even 'paternalism' (the very thing autonomy was meant to guard against) in a way that takes account of the actual reality for people with severe dementia. The advance directive will be relevant to these three further principles, but not – from the ethical perspective – as a non-negotiable legal dictate.

The case of futility

Turning to the issue of resuscitation (see case study), all hospital trusts in the UK should now have resuscitation policies, which tend to state that, unless a decision not to resuscitate has been properly made, resuscitation should take place. In which case, Mrs Timms should be resuscitated. But is this right? The risks attached to cardiopulmonary resuscitation (CPR) make this an important ethical decision (van Delden, 2000). The risk of fracturing the ribs of frail Mrs. Timms is real. The ethical debate here is often couched in terms of futility.

Case study: Mrs Timms

Mrs Timms was an 82-year-old lady admitted to the Elderly Severely Mentally Infirm (ESMI) Unit with a severe dementia. She had lost language and required feeding, help with dressing, toileting and personal hygiene. Initially she was mobile and wandered incessantly around the corridors. After a few months she became immobile. A niece visited her weekly. Over the course of 2 years she lost weight and spent more time sleeping. She was on little medication, for constipation, hypertension and heart failure. She became more frail. One morning the nurse went into her room and found her warm, but not breathing and with no pulse. Should the nurse commence cardiopulmonary resuscitation (CPR)?

Claims about futility are typically quantitative. For example, 'If it doesn't work for the last 100 patients, it is futile to try it on the next one'.

However, such claims cannot escape some form of qualitative statement too. For example, 'If the patient doesn't appreciate the benefit, it's futile' (Schneiderman and Jecker, 1995).

There are (quantitative) arguments about whether or not being old itself makes CPR futile. There may be characteristics that make CPR ineffective in older people (Murphy et al, 1989). It has to be recognized that CPR is not terribly effective under the best of conditions, let alone on a dementia unit (Awoke et al, 1992). And there is good evidence that the chances of survival after CPR in people with dementia is almost as poor as it is for people with metastatic cancer (Ebell et al, 1998).

Despite this quantitative evidence, however, it is still possible for someone to argue that resuscitation would be valuable in the next person with dementia. In fact, it is our experience that some carers do argue thus, even if they mostly

---

Table 4.1: Reaching decisions on resuscitation

For patients with severe dementia who have been admitted to a dementia unit where resuscitation has not previously been discussed:

- Nursing assessment involves judgements about the person's quality of life based on his or her current physical and mental health
- Learning more about the person's history will include learning about his or her previous values
- This enables a sensitive discussion to take place between the key nurse and the main carer
- Discussion of the issues involved may turn out to be too distressing or burdensome for the main carer
- A multidisciplinary decision should be reached involving the senior doctor, the key nurse, the main carers (to the extent that they are willing and able to participate) and any others involved in the person's care
- The nature, purpose and likely outcome of CPR need to be fully understood by those involved in the decision
- It is appropriate to consider not resuscitating if:
  1. CPR is unlikely to be successful (see discussion in Chapter 3)
  2. CPR is not in accord with the person's advance directive
  3. Successful CPR is likely to be followed by a length and quality of life that are judged not to be in the person's best interests

(British Medical Association, Resuscitation Council (UK) and Royal College of Nursing, 1999)

---

agree with decisions not to resuscitate (*Table 4.1*). Nevertheless, people usually do not use the futility argument to justify decisions not to resuscitate; rather they tend to point to the person's quality of life (which is discussed in Chapter 8) as being poor.

The trouble with the notion of 'futility' is that it sounds too harsh (Gillon, 1997). It does not resonate with the ethics of care, where the principles of protective responsibility, narrative integrity and candour seem more harmonious. On these grounds the nurse should not try to resuscitate Mrs Timms. Candour might suggest that the attempt to do so would be futile, but it also suggests that the appropriate decision, involving Mrs Timms's niece, should have been made so that the nurse was not left in the unenviable position of, in effect, trying to resuscitate a corpse purely to accord with the local resuscitation policy.

Similarly, protective responsibility and narrative integrity, over against futility, allow that how we treat Mrs Timms at the very end of her life should involve us taking the broadest possible view of her as a person (Hughes, 2001). This perspective allows that in some other case, where the person is alert and demonstrably happy, despite the statistics favouring futility, some form of resuscitation might perhaps be appropriate.

Ordinary and extraordinary treatments

*'Respect for life gives security to everyone in society. It respects
the whole bodily existence, yet accepts the inevitability of death. It
takes this reality and concludes that it is absolutely essential for the
good of humankind that no person's life, whatever their disability, is
declared to be useless. At the same time, it concludes that striving
to maintain life in certain circumstances may not be appropriate.
These circumstances occur when there is disproportion between the
treatment and its results, whether this is caused by ineffectiveness or
its burden.' (Jeffery, 2001)*

This is a recent statement of the distinction between ordinary and
extraordinary means, used by Catholic moral thinkers to justify the requirement
that treatments should be given under certain circumstances but not necessarily
under others. In fact, it is not only the Catholic church that recognizes that
extraordinary measures might be withheld in terminal care (Volicer, 1986).

Case study: Dr Brown

Dr Brown was a retired physician who had been receiving dialysis for many
years prior to his dementia. His dementia was now severe. Treatment of his
kidney failure was becoming more difficult. The kidney unit raised the question
of whether it was worth continuing treatment, when there were other people
who needed dialysis and would arguably benefit to a far greater extent. Was it
right to withdraw treatment, which would lead to Dr Brown's death, in order to
allow others to live longer or fuller lives?

In the case of Dr Brown, we can imagine that when his dementia was only
mild it seemed right to continue the treatment of his renal failure. When his
dementia became severe, however, it became more and more of a burden for him
to receive dialysis: not only did he no longer understand what was occurring, but
his distress at the treatment and his attempts to pull out the tubes required for
dialysis made the whole procedure too burdensome. To enforce such treatment
would seem extraordinary and, as such, without moral necessity or justification.

This helps to stress that it is not the treatment itself, or lack of it, that
is considered ordinary or extraordinary, but the treatment relevant to the
concrete circumstances of the case. Earlier chapters have considered treatment
of infections in dementia. In some circumstances treatment with antibiotics
might seem ordinary enough; while in other circumstances – if, for instance,
intravenous antibiotics were required – treatment might seem too burdensome
and thus extraordinary (Potkins et al, 2000). Similarly for issues around
feeding, it may seem ordinary in some circumstances to use tube feeding (e.g.
after some strokes) but extraordinary in others (e.g. in the terminal phases of
severe dementia) (Hughes, 2002).

The difficulty is that views vary. Several studies have demonstrated differences between carers and clinicians (Coetzee et al, 2003; Moe and Schroll, 1997). What would be useful would be further qualitative studies to try to understand the motivation behind the different views. Perhaps carers and clinicians are aiming at the same thing, but differ in terms of their perspectives on how burdensome a treatment might be. Still, any characterization of the ethics of care (see Chapter 2) tends to emphasize the concrete circumstances of particular cases, and it is in this context that talk of ordinary and extraordinary makes some sense.

Ethics and euthanasia

The principle of double effect depends on a distinction between foreseeing and intending an outcome. It is moral, according to this doctrine, to give Miss Schmall medication that might shorten her life if (and only if) the intention is to ease her pain (see case study). There is a tendency among clinicians to support the notion of double effect. There is no type of treatment that does not involve side-effects and, although clinicians can foresee the possibility of such side-effects, none (unless malicious) intends their patients to suffer adverse effects (albeit there may be intended beneficial side-effects) (Gillon, 1999).

Case study: Miss Schmall

Miss Schmall had a moderately severe dementia as well as known cancer when she was admitted very confused to the dementia unit. She seemed to accept her new surroundings without question. At times she had severe pains. She was prescribed high doses of both sedatives and analgesics. One of the nursing team expressed unease about the purpose and safety of these dosages and omitted the analgesia. However, the patient was very soon unable to sleep because of extreme pain. The case was discussed within the nursing team. More experienced members of the team argued that the purpose of the high doses of medication was to overcome the pain and not to shorten life. The person's life expectancy was measured in weeks rather than months. Even if the large doses of medication had foreseeable adverse effects, the risks involved to ensure adequate analgesia seemed reasonable. The intention was not to shorten Miss Schmall's life but to minimize her pain. She died a few days later having gone to lie on her bed for a rest after lunch. She had muttered about 'a bit of indigestion' before falling asleep and dying.

On the other hand, ethicists tend to dispute the doctrine, saying that the distinctions it draws are too difficult to specify exactly (Glover, 1977), or rely too much on the character of the clinicians, who have to distinguish between what they foresee and what they intend (Doyal, 1999).

One possible response to these objections is again to point to the broader context within which such decisions are made. It matters little what was going on in my mind (whether I thought I was foreseeing or intending) as I administered a lethal medication. Such a medication, by its nature, aims at killing the patient and this aim specifies the intention embodied in the action. It is not simply a foreseen consequence: the only possible outcome of giving a lethal injection (barring a mishap) is that it should be lethal. And this is not characteristically what is going on when a doctor treats a patient, even when the patient dies.

But perhaps the doctor should aim at the death of the patient. Euthanasia is either active or passive, depending on whether the death is brought about deliberately or simply allowed to happen. An injection of potassium chloride would be an active killing, whereas withholding food and fluid would be a passive way to end the person's life. This distinction may or may not be of moral significance: it is the difference between acts and omissions (Hope et al, 2003). Some argue that we can be held responsible for our acts, but that we are less morally culpable for our omissions. To kill someone by doing something to them might be wrong, but to allow them to die through withholding treatment is to allow nature to take its course, for which we cannot be held responsible.

Euthanasia is also split into voluntary (where the person seeks their death), involuntary (where they do not wish to die) and non-voluntary (where they are not competent to express their preferences, or perhaps have none) (Grey, 2000). Some pressure groups want active voluntary euthanasia to be legalized, so that competent people can stipulate when they want to die.

At the other extreme is active involuntary euthanasia, where people with no wish to die are killed, as in the Nazi death camps. In the case of dementia, we are normally talking about non-voluntary euthanasia. In passive non-voluntary euthanasia people are allowed to die because treatments are not given. Active non-voluntary euthanasia would involve the intentional killing of people with dementia on the grounds that, for instance, their quality of life was negligible.

Space does not allow us to discuss these issues in depth. There are, however, texts that pursue the arguments on either side in great detail (Keown, 1995). Rather than rehearse these arguments, we would wish to conclude with a thought, couched in the terms used by virtue ethicists.

Virtue ethics suggests that an action is right inasmuch as it is the action that the virtuous person would pursue. Virtue ethics, therefore, focuses attention on the character of the person doing or not doing whatever it is. In this way it suggests that what we become by our actions, or by our inaction, is relevant to whether or not the action is right or wrong. Hence, what do we *become* by caring for some of the most dependent members of our society? Or, what do we *become* by aiming at the death of the same people?

If we are allowed to kill people with dementia, without their consent or even with it, we are changed as people and as professionals. Our inclination is to lay greater emphasis on the need for appropriate resources and structures to encourage palliative care for people with dementia. Active non-voluntary euthanasia gets rid of a burden that faces society, but does not allow the sort of personal growth that caring for someone with dementia often allows. To deny this possibility is to deny the possibility of humans flourishing through sensitive communication, deep concern and intimacy.

In brief, before concluding, the argument in favour of killing people with dementia (whether or not they have asked to be killed) often relies upon the thought that they are suffering unbearably. (This is central to the Dutch legislation that allows euthanasia for people able to consent to it.) Euthanasia then seems to be a matter of caring. The problem with this argument is that it places too great an emphasis on whatever it is that people say to themselves to justify their actions. Of course, what we say to ourselves is important, but the possibility of self-deception is real. A counter argument is that the action itself has to be judged. Once this is seen to be an act of intentional killing, the justification for it becomes more problematic. These arguments would need more space than we have, but it is easy enough to see why the Select Committee on Medical Ethics, set up by the House of Lords, described the 'prohibition of intentional killing' as 'the cornerstone of law and of social relationships' (House of Lords, 1994). Our argument, in turn, is that the virtues implicit in caring are properly manifest only when human life itself is regarded as a good. But where the intentional killing of human life is allowed, this cannot be the case. Faced by unbearable suffering, therefore, genuine care would look towards palliative care rather than euthanasia, even if palliative care (at – but only at – the extreme) required complete sedation.

Conclusion

In discussing end-of-life ethical issues we have tended to stress the importance of the concrete complexity of individual cases. In the context of such cases we can usually find some form of consensus concerning what is right and what is wrong.

The application of principles and doctrines must in the end be justified by some broader notion of what is good or bad for humankind. One way to conceive this is in terms of the virtues: those dispositions that contribute to human flourishing, which determine how we become better human beings. In our view, palliative care for people with dementia, rather than having them killed, is a better way of demonstrating our humanity.

References

Agich GJ (2003) *Dependence and Autonomy in Old Age: An Ethical Framework for Long-Term Care*. 2nd edn. Cambridge University Press, Cambridge: 125

Awoke S, Mouton CP, Parrott M (1992) Outcomes of skilled cardiopulmonary resuscitation in a long-term-care facility: futile therapy? *J Am Geriatr Soc* **40**(6): 593–5

Beauchamp TL, Childress JF (2001) *Principles of Biomedical Ethics*. 5th edn. Oxford University Press, New York

British Medical Association, Resuscitation Council (UK) and the Royal College of Nursing (1999) Decisions relating to cardiopulmonary resuscitation. In: *J Med Ethics* (2001) **27**: 310–16

Coetzee RH, Leask SJ, Jones RG (2003) The attitudes of carers and old age psychiatrists towards the treatment of potentially fatal events in end-stage dementia. *Int J Geriatr Psychiatry* **18**(2): 169–173

Doyal L (1999) When doctors might kill their patients. The moral character of clinicians or the best interests of patients? *Br Med J* **318**(7196): 1432–3

Ebell MH, Becker LA, Barry HC, Hagen M (1998) Survival after in-hospital cardiopulmonary resuscitation. A meta-analysis. *J Gen Intern Med* **13**(12): 805–16

Gillon R (1997) 'Futility' – too ambiguous and pejorative a term? *J Med Ethics* 23(6): 339–40

Gillon R (1999) When doctors might kill their patients. Foreseeing is not necessarily the same as intending. *Br Med J* **318**(7196): 1431–2

Glover J (1977) *Causing Death and Saving Lives*. Penguin, Harmondsworth: 86–91

Grey W (2000) Right to die or duty to live? The problem of euthanasia. In: Dickenson D, Johnson M, Katz JS (eds) *Death, Dying and Bereavement*. Open University and Sage, London: 270–83

Hope T, Savulescu J, Hendrick J (2003) *Medical Ethics and Law: The Core Curriculum*. Churchill Livingstone, Edinburgh: 157–75

House of Lords (1994) *Report of the Select Committee on Medical Ethics*. Papers 21-I of 1993-94. HMSO, London: paragraph 237

Hughes JC (2001) Views of the person with dementia. *J Med Ethics* **27**(2): 86–91

Hughes JC (2002) Ethics and the psychiatry of old age. In: Jacoby R, Oppenheimer C (eds) *Psychiatry in the Elderly*. 3rd edn. Oxford University Press, Oxford: 863–895

Hughes JC, Louw SJ (2005) Moral, ethical and legal aspects of dementia: end-of-life decisions. In: Burns A, O'Brien J, Ames D (eds) *Dementia*. 3rd edn. Arnold Health Sciences, London: 239-43

Jeffery P (2001) *Going Against the Stream: Ethical Aspects of Ageing and Care*. Gracewing, Leominster (UK) and Liturgical Press, Collegeville (USA): 179

Keown J (ed) (1995) *Euthanasia Examined: Ethical, Clinical and Legal Perspectives*. Cambridge University Press, Cambridge

Lord Chancellor's Department (1997) *Who Decides? Making Decisions on Behalf of Mentally Incapacitated Adults*. HMSO, London

Moe C, Schroll M (1997) What degree of medical treatment do nursing home residents want in case of life-threatening disease? *Age Ageing* **26**(2): 133–137

Murphy DJ, Murray AM, Robinson BE, Campion EW (1989) Outcomes of cardiopulmonary resuscitation in the elderly. *Ann Intern Med* **111**(3): 199–205

Potkins D, Bradley S, Shrimanker J et al (2000) End of life treatment decisions in people with dementia: carers' views and the factors which influence them. *Int J Geriatr Psychiatry* **15**(11): 1005–8

Schneiderman LJ, Jecker NS (1995) *Wrong Medicine: Doctors, Patients, and Futile Treatment*. Johns Hopkins University Press, Baltimore and London

Vallis J, Boyd K (2002) Ethics and end-of-life decision-making. In: Hockley J, Clark D (eds) *Palliative Care for Older People in Care Homes*. Open University Press, Buckingham and Philadelphia: 120–37

van Delden JJM (2000) Do-not-resuscitate decisions. In: Dickenson D, Johnson M, Katz JS (eds) *Death, Dying and Bereavement*. Open University and Sage, London: 240–9

Volicer L (1986) Need for hospice approach to treatment of patients with advanced progressive dementia. *J Am Geriatr Soc* **34**(9): 655–8

Key points

- Advance directives, resuscitation decisions, what might be disproportionate treatment and intentions, all need to be broadly interpreted in concrete circumstances.

- The principles of medical ethics need to be augmented in dementia care by other principles that emphasize relationships, dependency and narrative.

- Virtue ethics stresses what we become by doing or not doing things.

- Providing good quality palliative care in dementia is a way of flourishing humanly.

Chapter 5

Different forms of psychological interventions in dementia

Ian James, Simon Douglas, Clive Ballard

In recent years there has been an increasing trend towards new conceptualizations of dementia that avoid the rather narrow frame of reference of the biomedical disease model (Bond, 2001). For example, Kitwood (1997) viewed dementia from a psychological perspective, with a focus on the 'personhood' of the individual with dementia and explored new ways of enhancing his or her 'quality of life'.

This has opened up new therapeutic options in the care and treatment of people with dementia, particularly with regard to psychological therapies. In fact, the use of these therapies has recently been recommended as a first-line treatment for people with the disease (Howard et al, 2001).

There is an increasing number of psychological therapies now available for people with dementia. As described by Ballard et al (2001), these therapies overlap and, in fact, individual approaches are rarely used in isolation. It is important, therefore, for clinicians to be familiar with a number of approaches in order to tailor combinations of treatment to the individual requirements of the person with dementia. Moreover, used in this way, psychological therapies square with many of the features of palliative care (i.e. affirming life, relieving distress, being holistic and involving families); thus, psychological approaches provide some validity for the use of the palliative care approach in dementia (as described in Chapter 1).

It is helpful to distinguish between two different forms of intervention. The first is a general or 'non-specific' type designed to promote a positive therapeutic milieu and positive wellbeing in people with dementia. The second is more problem-focused. In the latter case, typically a difficulty has already been diagnosed (e.g. depression, anxiety) or observed (e.g. agitation, shouting, wandering) and the intervention is specifically targeted at the problem or its causes.

These interventions routinely involve the development of a formulation to help understand the triggering and maintaining features of the problem. The goal of the formulation is to obtain an understanding of the 'needs' underpinning the 'challenging behaviour' (Cohen-Mansfield et al, 1997). For example: Is Mr B. shouting because he is communicating his pain? Is Mrs D. parcelling and hiding faeces because of her inability to locate the toilet and her resulting embarrassment. This chapter will examine both types of intervention separately, and reflect on the overlap between them (*Tables 5.1 and 5.2*).

Table 5.1: Non-specific psychological interventions

Standard interventions

- Reality orientation is one of the most widely-used management strategies for dealing with people with dementia. It aims to help people with memory loss and disorientation by reminding them of facts about themselves and their environment
- Validation therapy attempts to communicate with the person with dementia by empathizing with the feelings and hidden meanings behind his or her confused speech and behaviour. It is the emotional content of what is being said that is, therefore, more important than the person's orientation to the present
- Reminiscence therapy involves assisting the person with dementia to relive past experiences, especially those that might be positive and personally significant, such as family holidays or weddings. Group sessions tend to use activities such as art or music, and often use artefacts to provide stimulation.

Non-standard (alternative) interventions

- Art therapy has been recommended as a treatment for people with dementia as it has the potential to provide meaningful stimulation, improve social interaction and improve levels of self-esteem (Killick and Allan, 1999)
- Music therapy may involve the person engaging in a musical activity, or merely listening to songs or compositions
- Activity therapy is a rather amorphous group of behaviours such as dance, sport, drama, etc – all aimed at improving or maintaining general health
- Other complementary therapies: e.g. herbal medicine, massage, reflexology and therapeutic healing, for which there is generally little empirical evidence. However, there is more evidence in favour of aromatherapy, bright light therapy and multisensory approaches
- Aromatherapy: the two main essential oils used in aromatherapy for dementia are extracted from lavender and melissa balm. They have the advantage that there are several routes of administration such as inhalation, bathing or massage, or topical application in a cream
- Bright light therapy probably works through its effects on the sleep–wake cycle
- Multisensory approaches: e.g. use of a Snoezelen room with various smells and sounds, lights (flexible fibre optics) and textures.
- Doll therapy is a controversial intervention, involving giving people with dementia the opportunity to take ownership of a doll.

Table 5.2: Non-specific psychological interventions

- Behaviour therapy
- Cognitive behaviour therapy (CBT)
- Interpersonal therapy (IPT).

Non-specific psychological interventions

This form of intervention is designed to create an atmosphere and environment that will promote the positive wellbeing of people with dementia. Many of the interventions in this category could be termed person-centred (Kitwood, 1997) since they are designed

1. To focus on a person's strengths
2. To support the person in difficulty
3. To foster psychological health and validate daily experiences.

In this section, the non-specific interventions will be described in terms of standard versus non-standard treatments. The standard approaches are considered to be the more established and empirically tested interventions, while the non-standard ones are often regarded as 'alternative' therapies.

Standard interventions

Reality orientation
Although not usually regarded as a person-centred approach, when used appropriately, reality orientation helps the person re-orientate him or herself in a validating way. For example, through helping a man to accept that he is actually 75 years' old and retired with a large family, one is then able to cue him into searching for positive and validating memories about his previous work, his children, and the joys of grandparenthood.

There has been debate regarding the efficacy of the approach, with concern that it might remind people of their deterioration, or be too confrontational. However, a recent review of the six randomized-controlled trials available was favourable (Spector et al, 2002a).

Validation therapy
Naomi Feil, the originator of validation therapy, suggested that some of the features associated with dementia, such as repetition and retreating into the past, were in fact active strategies on the part of the person with dementia

to avoid stress, boredom and loneliness (Feil, 1993). She argued that people with dementia can retreat into an inner reality based on feelings rather than intellect as they find the present reality too painful. Neal and Briggs (2002) evaluated validation therapy's effectiveness across a number of controlled trials, employing cognitive and behavioural measures. They concluded that despite some positive indicators, the jury was still out with respect to its efficacy.

Reminiscence therapy
Spector et al (2002b) identified only two randomized controlled trials of reminiscence therapy. Based on their limited data set they concluded that there was little evidence of a significant impact of the approach. However, O'Donovan (1993) stated that while there is little indication of cognitive improvements, there is some evidence suggesting improvements in behaviour, wellbeing, social and self-care, and motivation (Baines et al, 1987; Gibson, 1994; Brooker 2001).

It is claimed that pre-morbid aspects of the person's personality may re-emerge during reminiscence work (Woods, 1999). The therapy has a great deal of flexibility as it can be adapted to the individual with dementia. A person with severe dementia can still gain pleasure from listening to an old record, for instance.

Non-standard interventions

In the current context, this group of interventions is frequently viewed as 'alternative' therapies. As in other areas of health care, alternative therapies are gaining currency in the treatment of people with dementia. These therapies still often lack empirical evidence relating to their efficacy, but this issue is gradually being addressed. A review of the most popular forms of therapy is provided below.

Art therapy
This can involve the person drawing and painting, which is seen to provide him or her with the opportunity for self-expression and the chance to exercise some choice in terms of colours or theme of picture (Killick and Allan, 1999).

Music therapy
Several studies have reported benefits gained by people with dementia from music therapy (Casby and Holm, 1994). For example, Lord and Garner (1993) recorded increases in levels of wellbeing, better social interaction and improvements in autobiographical memory in a group of nursing home residents who were played music. Such improvements were not observed in a comparison group engaged in other activities.

Activity therapy
It has been shown that physical exercise can have a number of health benefits for people with dementia, reducing falls, improving mental health and sleep, decreasing night-time agitation, improving mood and confidence.

Complementary therapy
The Mental Health Foundation conducted a study into the use of complementary therapies in the field of mental health (Wallcraft, 1998), including their use with people with dementia. From this work it was evident that a number of different therapies were being employed, such as massage, reflexology, therapeutic healing, herbal medicine and aromatherapy (Wiles and Brooker, 2003). In general, most of the complementary therapies have not received a great deal of empirical investigation. An exception to this is aromatherapy.

Aromatherapy
This is one of the fastest growing of all the complementary therapies (Burns et al, 2002). It appears to have several advantages over the widely-used pharmacological treatments in dementia. It has a positive image and its use aids interaction while providing a sensory experience. It also seems to be well tolerated in comparison to neuroleptic or other sedative medication. There have been some positive results from recent controlled trials which have shown significant improvements in agitation symptoms with excellent compliance and tolerability (Ballard et al, 2002).

Bright light therapy
Recent controlled trials using bright light therapy have been published with some evidence for improving restlessness but with particular benefit for sleep disturbances (Graf et al, 2001; Haffmans et al, 2001).

Multisensory approaches
These typically involve a Snoezelen room in which multisensory stimulation is provided often in a non-directive and failure-free environment. Recent studies show positive, though not conclusive, effects for the therapy (Baillon et al, 2004).

Doll therapy
There is a great deal of anecdotal evidence of the benefits of providing dolls to people with dementia (Godfrey, 1994; Ehrenfeld and Bergman, 1995). It is only recently, however, that it has been explored more formally in homes for the Elderly Mentally Infirm (EMI) (Mackenzie et al, 2005). Mackenzie's pilot study showed improvements in behaviour, affect and levels of staff-resident interaction, following the introduction of dolls. In addition to the obvious ethical problems associated with such an approach (Cayton, 2006), practical problems were also identified in the pilot study. For example, residents argued over the ownership of dolls.

Problem-specific interventions

In this section we describe interventions that specifically target client or resident problems that have been either identified or diagnosed. The interventions involve the development of formulations to help those involved to understand what triggers and maintains the difficulties for the person with dementia (Stokes, 2000).

Behaviour therapy

Traditionally, behaviour therapy has been based on principles of conditioning and learning theory using strategies aimed at suppressing or eliminating challenging behaviours. More recently, positive programming methodologies (La Vigna and Donnellan, 1986) have employed non-aversive methods in helping to develop more functional behaviours. Moniz-Cook et al (1998) suggest that behaviour analysis is often the starting point of most other forms of therapeutic intervention in this area. Furthermore, they propose that modern behavioural approaches can be wholly consistent with person-centred care.

Behaviour therapy requires a detailed assessment period in which the triggers, behaviours and reinforcers – i.e. the antecedents and consequences (ABC) – are identified and their relationships made clear. The therapist will often use some kind of chart or diary to gather information about the manifestations of a behaviour and the sequence of actions leading up to it. Interventions are then based on the analysis of these results. Emerson (1998) suggests focusing on three key features when designing an intervention:

1. Taking account of a person's preferences
2. Changing the context in which the behaviour takes place
3. Using reinforcement strategies and schedules that reduce the behaviour.

The efficacy of behavioural therapy has been demonstrated in the context of dementia in only a small number of studies (Burgio and Fisher, 2000). For example, there is evidence of successful reductions in wandering, incontinence and other forms of stereotypical behaviours (Bakke, 1997; Woods, 1999).

The new psychotherapies

Over the last 10 years there has been an increasing interest in applying cognitive behaviour therapy (CBT) and interpersonal therapy (IPT) to the area. It is relevant to note that these approaches often do not address the target problem (e.g. depression, agitation) directly. Indeed, they are helpful because they help professionals and carers to understand why the problems are arising and how they are being maintained. Once this has been done, more often than not, very practical interventions are used to intervene.

The case study below demonstrates how the CBT framework can encourage a formulation that allows a greater understanding of the 'problem' behaviour and thereby opens up ways to help the person rather than just treat the symptom.

Case study: Mrs Gilligan

Mrs Gilligan, who lived in a nursing home, was referred because of her wandering and 'disruptive screaming'. Using a CBT framework (James 1999a;b), it was discovered that she had a chronic history of post-traumatic stress disorder (caused by a violent burglary). Hence, it was determined that her shouting at night was the result of flashbacks to the burglary rather than being any form of 'attention seeking' behaviour. The practical intervention derived from the CBT framework simply involved relocating her to a shared room where she felt more secure. This approach was in stark contrast to the previous strategy, which involved placing her at the far end of the ward by herself so that she would not disturb the other residents.

IPT, as the name suggests, examines the person's distress within an interpersonal context. It uses a specific framework whereby a person's distress is conceptualized through one of four domains:

1. Interpersonal disputes
2. Interpersonal/personality difficulties
3. Bereavement
4. Transitions/life events.

Despite there being good empirical evidence for this form of treatment with older people (Miller and Reynolds, 2002), it has only recently been applied to the area of dementia (James et al, 2003). With respect to both of these therapies there are limitations to using such approaches, particularly with those with severe dementia. Nevertheless, because these therapies have relatively simple conceptual models underpinning them, they have been shown to be helpful – even when working with people with severe cognitive impairment (James, 1999a;b).

Conclusion

Having reviewed many of the treatments currently available, it is worth noting the commonalities between the various interventions. One striking thing is the general move towards a more person-centred focus of care (Kitwood,

1997). Within this form of care, greater attempts are made to understand the individual's experience of his or her dementia, and to employ strategies to improve the person's quality of life. This involves the acknowledgement of the person's view of reality and the fact that he or she has feelings, emotions and the ability to live in relationships (Bond, 2001).

It is this ability that leads to a further shared feature of these interventions: their systemic perspective. It is important to recognize how the context of a person with dementia's relationships with family and caregivers affects both the individual with dementia and his or her caregivers. Such a view emphasizes the need to work with all of the systems involved in the person's care (families, professional carers, organizations etc.). Indeed, care staff and families are usually integral to treatment strategies and are essential in obtaining valid and reliable information and constructing appropriate formulations. Also, they are key to conducting the intervention reliably.

It is evident, therefore, that carer or staff training and support is a crucial part of most treatment programmes. However, despite recognition of this issue in the literature, there remain relatively few quality studies (Cohen-Mansfield et al, 1997; Moniz-Cook et al, 1998; Proctor et al, 1999). Clearly it is an important area worthy of further study.

References

Baillon S, Van Diepen E, Prettyman R et al (2004) A comparison of the effects of Snoezelen and reminiscence therapy on the agitated behaviour of patients with dementia. *Int J Geriat Psychiatry* **19**(11): 1047-1052

Baines S, Saxby P, Ehlert K (1987) Reality orientation and reminiscence therapy: a controlled cross-over study of elderly confused people. *Brit J Psychiatry* **151**(Aug): 222–31

Bakke B (1997) Applied behaviour analysis for behavioural problems in Alzheimer's disease. *Geriatrics* **52**(suppl 12): 40–3

Ballard CG, O'Brien J, James I, Swann A (2001) *Dementia: Management of Behavioural and Psychological Symptoms*. Oxford University Press, Oxford

Ballard CG, O'Brien J, Reichelt K, Perry E (2002) Aromatherapy as a safe and effective treatment for the management of agitation in severe dementia: the results of a double-blind, placebo-controlled trial with melissa. *J Clin Psychiatry* **63**(7): 553–8

Bond J (2001) Sociological perspectives. In: Cantley C (ed) *A Handbook of Dementia Care*. Open University Press, Buckingham: 44–61

Brooker D (2001) Therapeutic activity. In: Cantley C (ed) *A Handbook of Dementia Care*. Open University Press, Buckingham: 146–59

Burgio L, Fisher S (2000) Application of psychosocial interventions for treating behavioural and psychological symptoms of dementia. *Int Psychogeriatr* **12**(Suppl 1): 351–8

Burns A, Byrne J, Ballard C, Holmes C (2002) Sensory stimulation in dementia: an effective option for managing behavioural problems. *Br Med J* **325**(7376): 1312–3

Casby J, Holm M (1994) The effect of music on repetitive disruptive vocalizations of persons with dementia. *Am J Occup Ther* **48**(10): 883–9

Cayton H (2006) From childhood to childhood? Autonomy and dependence through the ages of life. In Hughes JC, Louw SJ, Sabat SR (eds) *Dementia: Mind, Meaning, and the Person*. Oxford University Press, Oxford: 277–86.

Cohen-Mansfield J, Werner P, Culpepper WJ, Barkley D (1997) Evaluation of an in-service training programme on dementia and wandering. *J Gerontol Nurs* **23**(10): 40–7

Ehrenfeld M, Bergman R (1995) The therapeutic use of dolls. *Perspect Psychiatr Care* **31**(4): 21-22

Emerson E (1998) Working with people with challenging behaviour. In: Emerson E, Hatton C, Bromley J, Caine A (eds) *Clinical Psychology and People with Intellectual Disabilities*. John Wiley & Sons, Chichester: 127–53.

Feil N (1993) *The Validation Breakthrough: Simple Techniques for Communicating with People with 'Alzheimer's-Type Dementia'*. Health Professions Press, Baltimore, MD

Gibson F (1994) What can reminiscence contribute to people with dementia? In: Bornat J (ed) *Reminiscence Reviewed: Evaluations, Achievements, Perspectives*. Open University Press, Buckingham: 46–60

Godfrey S (1994) Doll therapy. *Aust J Ageing* **13**(1): 46

Graf A, Wallner C, Schubert V (2001) The effects of light therapy on mini-mental state examination scores in demented patients. *Biol Psychiatry* **50**(9): 725 7

Haffmans PM, Sival RC, Lucius SA et al (2001) Bright light therapy and melatonin in motor restless behaviour in dementia: a placebo-controlled study. *Int J Geriat Psychiatry* **16**(1): 106–10

Howard R, Ballard C, O'Brien J, Burns A (2001) UK and Ireland Group for optimization of management in dementia. Guidelines for the management of agitation in dementia. *Int J Geriat Psychiatry* **16**(7): 714–7

James I (1999a) Using a cognitive rationale to conceptualise anxiety in people with dementia. *Behav Cogn Psychother* **27**(4): 345–51

James I (1999b) Cognitive conceptualisation of distress in dementia. *Clin Psychol Forum* **133**(Nov): 21–5

James IA, Postma K, Mackenzie L (2003) Using an IPT conceptualisation to treat a depressed person with dementia. *Behav Cogn Psychother* **31**(4): 451–6

Killick J, Allan K (1999) The arts in dementia care: tapping a rich resource. *J Dementia Care* **7**(4): 35–8

Kitwood T (1997) *Dementia Reconsidered: The Person Comes First*. Open University Press, Buckingham

La Vigna G, Donnellan A (1986) *Alternative to Punishment: Solving Behavior Problems with Non-aversive Strategies*. Irvington, New York

Lord T, Garner E (1993) Effects of music on Alzheimer patients. *Percep Mot Skills* **76**(2): 451–5

Mackenzie L, James IA, Morse R (2005) *A pilot study on the use of dolls on people with dementia*. National PSIGE conference, British Psychological Society, Chester. Paper and poster presentations. Contact address: Centre for the Health of the Elderly, Newcastle General Hospital, Newcastle upon Tyne, NE4 6BE

Miller M, Reynolds C (2002) Interpersonal psychotherapy. In: Hepple J, Pearce J, Wilkinson P (eds) *Psychological Therapies With Older People: Developing Treatments for Effective Practice*. Bruner-Routledge, Sussex: 103–27

Moniz-Cook E, Agar S, Silver M et al (1998) Can staff training reduce behavioural problems in residential care for the elderly mentally ill? *Int J Geriat Psychiatry* **13**(3): 149–58

Neal M, Briggs M (2002) Validation therapy for dementia (Cochrane review). In: *The Cochrane Library*. Issue 2. John Wiley & Sons, Chichester, UK

O'Donovan S (1993) The memory lingers on. *Nurs Elder* **5**(1): 27–31

Proctor R, Burns A, Powell H et al (1999) Behavioural management in nursing and residential homes: a randomised control trial. *Lancet* **354**(9172): 26–9

Stokes G (2000) *Challenging Behaviour in Dementia*. Speechmark, Bicester

Spector A, Orrell M, Davies S, Woods B (2002a) Reality orientation for dementia (Cochrane review). In: *Cochrane Library*. Issue 2. John Wiley & Sons, Chichester

Spector A, Orrell M, Davies S, Woods RT (2002b) Reminiscence therapy for dementia (Cochrane review). In Cochrane Library. Issue 2. John Wiley & Sons, Chichester

Wallcraft J (1998) *Healing Minds*. Mental Health Foundation, London

Wiles A, Brooker D (2003) Complementary therapies in dementia care. *J Dementia Care* **11**(3): 31–6

Woods RT (1999) *Psychological Problems of Ageing*. John Wiley and Sons, Chichester

Key points

- Psychological therapies are recommended as first-line treatments for people with dementia.

- Psychological therapies can claim to be person-centred by allowing a flexible approach based on an individual formulation.

- Non-specific therapies aim to promote a positive therapeutic milieu and wellbeing; problem-focused therapies look for factors that trigger and maintain a behaviour.

- Some psychological therapies have a good evidence base, but for other therapies the empirical evidence is lacking.

- The context of care may contribute to the problem behaviour, but may also provide a large part of the solution.

Chapter 6

Drugs used to relieve the behavioural symptoms of dementia

Clive Ballard, Lisa Hulford

Over 90% of people with dementia develop behavioural problems or psychiatric symptoms at some point during their illness (Ballard et al, 2001b). These disturbances are varied in their presentation and underlying aetiology and are collectively referred to as 'behavioural and psychological signs and symptoms of dementia' (BPSD) (Finkel et al, 1996). There are at least three distinct major BPSD:

- Psychotic symptoms (delusions and hallucinations)
- Mood disorder (depression, anxiety, apathy, hypomania)
- Agitation.

Agitation is the most frequent and disturbing of the BPSD in people with more severe dementia and among those living in nursing homes or residential care. The term 'agitation' is often misused, but correctly defined it describes a syndrome characterized by excessive motor activity and a feeling of inner tension, with a cluster of related symptoms including anxiety and irritability, motor restlessness and abnormal vocalization (e.g. shouting). BPSD represent a major source of stress and burden to family caregivers and precipitate institutionalization (Ballard et al, 2001b).

To inform treatment decisions, it is important to understand the natural course of these symptoms and their impact upon the individuals themselves. More than half of the individuals experiencing psychosis or depression will experience spontaneous resolution over a 3-month period, although agitation is likely to be more persistent (Ballard et al, 2001b). In addition, only a third of the individuals experiencing BPSD are distressed by the experience and these symptoms do not appear to have a detrimental impact upon the individual's quality of life (Ballard et al, 2001a).

These symptoms are, therefore, a potentially important treatment target, but in any individual situation it is important to determine whether the person experiencing the symptoms is distressed or at risk and whether there is a substantial impact upon others. If not, it will often be appropriate to monitor the situation rather than to treat automatically, particularly with pharmacotherapy.

Evidence-based guidelines for the management of BPSD have been developed in the UK and in Ireland (Howard et al, 2001). They recommend a full and careful assessment of the physical, psychological and environmental factors that might be of aetiological relevance and an assessment of the impact of the symptoms on other people, including an assessment of risk.

The quality of care available to the patient should be optimized to ensure that facilities and available skills meet the patient's needs. It is recommended that non-pharmacological management should be tried first and should be the mainstay of treatment (see Chapter 5). Pharmacological treatments are only indicated when other strategies have failed.

Drug therapies for treating symptoms of dementia

Major tranquillizers (neuroleptics or antipsychotics)

These drugs were originally developed to treat people with schizophrenia. At the moment, none of these treatments is specifically licensed to treat people with dementia, although they are frequently prescribed and are usually the first-line pharmacological treatment for BPSD.

In total, there are 15 published placebo-controlled studies examining the treatment of BPSD with neuroleptics (*Table 6.1*). Many of these studies are small, although four larger studies (three with risperidone, one with olanzapine) have been published over the past 5 years. It is convention to describe a good outcome as a 30% improvement on a standardized behavioural rating scale in these trials. Using this threshold, about 60% of people have had a good response to neuroleptics and 40% have had a good response to placebo across all the trials: a statistically significant but modest effect size (Ballard and O'Brien, 1999).

The results are difficult to interpret as the studies group together a range of dissimilar behavioural and psychiatric symptoms, which probably have different underlying aetiologies. A recent Cochrane review of haloperidol, for example, indicated that the evidence for efficacy was much stronger for the treatment of aggression than for other symptoms (Olin and Schneider, 2004). There is probably also a publication bias, as there are at least three unpublished studies (one each for risperidone, olanzapine and quetiapine) that have not shown significant benefit.

To inform treatment decisions, it is important to understand the timeframe of treatment response. The majority of trials focus on a treatment period of 4–12 weeks. They neither provide evidence of a significant improvement with single doses (hence the practice of 'as required' medication has no underpinning evidence), nor evidence of benefit over substantially longer treatment periods.

Table 6.1: Placebo-controlled trials of neuroleptics for behavioural symptoms

Study	Agent	Sample size	% Significantly improved vs placebo
Abse et al (1960)*	Chlorpromazine	32	No significant difference
Hamilton & Bennett (1962)*	Trifluoperazine	27	22% vs 0%
Hamilton & Bennett (1962)*	Acetophenazine	19	64% vs 20%
Sugarman et al (1964)*	Haloperidol	18	89% vs 67%
Cahn & Diestfeldt (1973)*	Penfluridol	36	No significant difference
Rada & Kellner (1976)*	Thiothixine	42	59% vs 55%
Petrie et al (1982)*	Haloperidol, loxapine	61	65% vs 58% vs 36%
Barnes et al (1982)*	Thioridazine, loxapine	53	59% vs 68% vs 47%
Finkel et al (1995)*	Thiothixene	33	65% vs 19%
Satterlee et al (1995)*	Olanzapine	238	No significant difference
Katz et al (1999)	Risperidone	435	68% vs 61%
De Deyn et al (1999)	Risperidone, haloperidol	344	76% vs 69% vs 61%
Teri et al (2000)	Haloperidol	149	32% vs 34%
Street et al (2000)	Olanzapine	206	65% vs 57% vs 43% vs 36%
Brodaty et al (2003)	Risperidone	301	Improvement: 13.5%>placebo

*Taken from Ballard and O'Brien, 1999

The latter is a concern since many people treated with these agents are prescribed them for a number of years.

Placebo-controlled withdrawal studies indicate that there is no worsening of behaviour when neuroleptic drugs are stopped (Cohen-Mansfield et al, 1999; Ballard et al, 2004). There is, therefore, very little evidence to support the practice of ongoing neuroleptic treatment. Prescriptions should be reviewed regularly and a trial discontinuation should probably be undertaken 3–6 months after the treatment is started.

The use of neuroleptics in people with dementia remains controversial because of the potentially harmful side effects and adverse outcomes (*Table 6.2*). In the UK, the Committee on Safety of Medicines (2004) has decided that risperidone

---

Table 6.2: Adverse effects of neuroleptics

- Excessive sedation
- Dizziness, unsteadiness and falls (often with associated injury such as fractures)
- Symptoms of Parkinson's disease (tremor, slowness and stiffness of the limbs)
- Severe sensitivity in people with dementia with Lewy bodies, possibly causing death in these individuals
- Increased risk of stroke with some drugs within this class, e.g. risperidone and olanzapine
- Changes in the electrocardiogram that may increase the risk of cardiac arrhythmias with some neuroleptics, e.g. thioridazine
- Evidence is also beginning to accumulate to suggest that neuroleptics may accelerate the rate of decline and disease progression in people with dementia; hence there are particular concerns over the long-term use of these drugs

---

and olanzapine should no longer be prescribed for the treatment of behavioural symptoms in people with dementia, because of the increased risk of stroke.

The higher risk of stroke with risperidone treatment was first described as part of a 12-week placebo-controlled trial of risperidone for the treatment of agitation in people with dementia (Brodaty et al, 2003). A subsequent analysis of this study and three other similar trials confirmed the higher risk of stroke. Based upon the evidence, for every year of treatment, between 1 in 4 and 1 in 14 people will have a stroke (who would not otherwise have had one) when treated with risperidone. Although there is less information available for olanzapine, as only two trials have been completed comparing olanzapine with a placebo in people with dementia, the risk appears to be similar (for details see Committee on Safety of Medicines, 2004).

A very recent study of the atypical antipsychotic quetiapine has shown that it has no benefit in patients with dementia and agitation (Ballard et al, 2005). This was a randomized double-blind placebo-controlled trial with 23 patients receiving the maximum protocol dose of quetiapine and 26 receiving placebo. More worryingly, quetiapine was associated with greater cognitive decline than placebo.

There is little doubt that neuroleptic drugs have *some* beneficial effects on behavioural disturbance in dementia. However, the benefits are limited and there is a substantial placebo effect. Moreover, this must be balanced against the high frequency of adverse effects.

It is, therefore, a cause of serious concern that more than one third of people with dementia in UK residential and nursing homes are prescribed neuroleptics, often without adequate monitoring. Many patients are clearly treated inappropriately with medication as a first-line treatment.

Anticonvulsant and antidepressant medication for agitation

Sodium valproate and carbamazepine, among others, are sometimes used to reduce aggression and agitation, as is the antidepressant drug trazodone. The best evidence for efficacy is for carbamazepine (Tariot et al, 1998, 1999), where two small placebo-controlled studies indicate benefit. However, adverse events, particularly unsteadiness and neutropenia (lowering of the white blood cells), are a cause for concern in older people.

Preliminary studies and a trial against a comparator drug suggest that trazodone may be useful (Sultzer et al, 1997), but the only placebo-controlled trial did not demonstrate significant efficacy (Teri et al, 2000). The study was small and probably lacked statistical power, and further work is still needed to determine whether trazodone has a useful place in the treatment of some BPSD. Notably, there is still no evidence from placebo-controlled trials that benzodiazepines (e.g. diazepam or lorazepam) are of value in BPSD, despite their widespread use.

Antidementia drugs: cholinesterase inhibitors

The new generation of anticholinesterase drugs (donepezil, rivastigmine, galantamine) were developed as symptomatic treatments for dementia and are licensed for the treatment of people with mild to moderate Alzheimer's disease. Preliminary evidence suggests that they may also have beneficial effects on behavioural symptoms.

Four of the studies (two with donepezil, two with galantamine) evaluating the benefits of these treatments on cognition and function have measured behaviour as a secondary outcome measure, with two of the four studies suggesting significant benefits (Birks and Harvey, 2004; Olin and Schneider, 2004). The symptoms most likely to improve appear to be apathy (lack of drive), mood, delusions and hallucinations. Most of these studies have focused on people with very low levels of behavioural disturbance and demonstrating reductions of 'behavioural scores' in these cohorts is not the same as demonstrating efficacy in people with clinically significant BPSD.

The results of ongoing studies evaluating this key question are still needed before the place of cholinesterase inhibitors in treating these symptoms is clear. One exception is the treatment of BPSD in people with dementia with Lewy bodies (characterized by the core features of fluctuating cognitive function, visual hallucinations and parkinsonism), where a placebo-controlled trial indicated significant benefits from rivastigmine treatment (Wild et al, 2004). Given the potential hazardous side effects of neuroleptics in these individuals, treatment with a cholinesterase inhibitor should probably be the first-line pharmacological intervention.

However, this conclusion must be tempered by the recent study (Ballard et al, 2005) that showed rivastigmine was of no benefit in comparison with a placebo group for patients with dementia and agitation in institutional care.

Antidementia drugs: memantine

Memantine is the most recently available antidementia drug and is licensed for the treatment of moderately-severe to severe Alzheimer's disease. It works in a different way to the anticholinesterase drugs, targeting a different type of nerve cell receptor (glutamate receptors). One preliminary report from a recent study indicates benefit for some behavioural symptoms (Cummings et al, 2004), including agitation, although a lot more work is needed to determine the potential benefits.

Drugs for treating depression

Symptoms of depression are common in dementia, occurring in approximately 20% of people with Alzheimer's disease and a higher proportion of people with vascular dementia or dementia with Lewy bodies (Ballard et al, 2001b). In Alzheimer's disease, two-thirds of people with depression experience spontaneous resolution of their symptoms over 3 months, although depression is more likely to be persistent in vascular dementia.

Ongoing depression is important, however. As well as the distress and health implications for the individual, it also has a substantial detrimental impact upon everyday activities and self-care. In early dementia, depression may be a reaction to the person's awareness of his or her diagnosis, or to life events. In the later stages of the illness, the environment remains very important but depression may also be the result of reduced chemical transmitter function in the brain. Simple non-drug interventions, such as an activity or exercise programme, can be very helpful (Douglas et al, 2004) and should probably be the first-line treatment for mild depression.

Tricyclic antidepressants (e.g. amitriptyline) are not appropriate for people with dementia as the cholinergic side effects are likely to worsen the severity of cognitive and functional impairments. There are relatively few placebo-controlled studies of other antidepressants with more favourable side effect profiles.

Two placebo-controlled trials with selective serotonin reuptake inhibitors (SSRIs) – with citalopram (Nyth and Gottfries, 1990) and sertraline (Lyketsos et al, 2003) – and one large trial with moclobemide (Roth et al, 1996), the reversible monoamine oxidase inhibitor, have demonstrated significant improvement in symptoms of depression in people with Alzheimer's disease.

In clinical practice, the pharmacological treatment of depression in the context of Alzheimer's disease should probably be focused on people with more severe symptoms (e.g. very poor appetite, decreased fluid intake, hopelessness, suicidal thoughts), individuals who are markedly distressed or experience increased functional impairments because of their depression, or when the symptoms are persistent.

One of the SSRI drugs, probably (in view of the trial evidence) sertraline or citalopram, is the treatment of choice. The optimal duration of therapy is unclear in the absence of any specific studies to inform practice, but treatment should probably be continued for at least 6 months after the resolution of symptoms and for a longer period if the depression has been recurrent. For milder or transient episodes of depression, non-pharmacological interventions are very effective (see Chapter 5).

The situation is slightly less clear for people who have vascular dementia, where the symptoms of depression are more frequent and more persistent. There are no trials specifically in people with vascular dementia, although trials in stroke patients have suggested that SSRIs are an effective treatment for depression in these individuals.

In practice, SSRIs are again probably the treatment of choice, but the threshold for preferring a pharmacological approach is lower in vascular dementia.

Summary

As June's case (below) shows, managing BPSD can be problematic. Drugs are useful, but they often have side effects. In practice, drugs are used empirically. Instead, the better approach is to take a broad view of the problems, without forgetting the possibility of pain or some other condition (such as an infection) causing a delirium (see Chapters 3 and 7). There should then be an attempt to treat BPSD as rationally as possible. This should involve an attempt to understand the behaviour, which in turn requires a formulation that encompasses the physical, psychological, social and spiritual dimensions of the person.

Case study: June

June is a woman in her late 70s suffering from severe dementia. She began to have slight memory problems several years ago. It was surmised that this was partly a consequence of a significant head injury when she was involved in a road traffic accident. Her memory impairment worsened following a series of small strokes and probably because of her high alcohol consumption.

Before the onset of her illness, June lived a happy and fulfilling life. She was married with three children and she worked as a school cleaner, moving with her family to live in Canada for several years. On returning to England, her husband developed Parkinson's disease and June became responsible for him. She also started drinking more heavily. Eventually, following the accident, her own problems meant that she had to be admitted to residential care when he went into a general nursing home. Her behaviour became difficult and she started to pose a risk to herself and to other people. She was admitted for assessment and then discharged to a NHS continuing care unit for people with severe dementia.

June now requires total nursing care because of her very poor mental functioning. She is extremely noisy and spends much of the day wandering around the unit shouting incoherently. She becomes very easily agitated and has a long history of violence and aggression, which is directed both at staff and family. She remains physically fit, fully ambulant and quite strong. As well as hitting, scratching and spitting, on more than one occasion she has been found attempting to strangle other immobile residents.

The aggressive behaviour has been very difficult to control with medication, because certain drugs have left her extremely sedated in a state that meant it was difficult to feed her. Having used a mixture of antidepressants, antipsychotics, benzodiazepines and mood-stabilizing drugs, the consultant in charge of her care instigated a low dose of morphine on the grounds that her distress might signal pain. The combination of a sedating antidepressant, a mood stabilizer and morphine appeared to lessen June's aggression, although some violence continues to be shown towards other people. Nevertheless, she appears to become tolerant to the medication and the doses of morphine have had to be increased. She is also prescribed diazepam and trazodone if required, although staff have found that this tends to upset her balance and increase the risk of her falling. Because of lack of staff, it has been difficult to manage June using more psychosocial approaches.

Discussion

June poses significant difficulties for the clinical team. The initial thought was that she might have been depressed and an antidepressant seemed a reasonable option. The antipsychotic was used for agitation, but despite raising the dose and giving the medication for at least 6 weeks, there were no benefits and increasing side effects. Benzodiazepines, chiefly lorazepam, were used when there were violent outbursts. Again, however, this made her more unsteady. The use of morphine produced a distinct improvement, but it is not entirely clear why: was she in pain, or has she benefited from its euphoric effects?

Reviewing the case history, it seems clearer that, on going into long-term care, June suffered significant losses. Her wandering could be interpreted as searching for her husband, for whom she had cared with devotion. The need for a more psychosocial approach seems clear. Perhaps June would benefit from a more soothing environment and more one-to-one time with her carers, being with her, rather than doing to her.

In brief, therefore, management of BPSD should keep in mind the following principles:

- Whenever possible, it is preferable to avoid additional drugs for people with dementia
- For most BPSD, non-pharmacological approaches are often effective and should be the first-line intervention
- For symptoms that are severe, distressing or put people at risk, pharmacological interventions can contribute to the management, although the potential benefits have to be weighed against the potential adverse effects
- These treatments should be reviewed regularly and stopped, either if they are ineffective or after an appropriate period of symptomatic resolution.

References

Ballard C, Margallo-Lana M, Juszczak E et al (2005) Quetiapine and Rivastigmine and cognitive decline in Alzheimer's disease: randomised double blind placebo controlled trial. *Br Med J Online* First bmj.com. BMJ, doi:10.1136/bmj.38369.459988.8F (published 18 February 2005) [Accessed 25 February 2005]

Ballard CG, O'Brien J (1999) Pharmacological treatment of behavioural and psychological signs in Alzheimer's disease: how good is the evidence for current pharmacological treatments? *Br Med J* **319**(7203): 18–9

Ballard C, O'Brien J, James I et al (2001a) Quality of life for people with dementia living in nursing home and residential care. *Int Psychogeriatr* **13**(1): 93–106

Ballard C, O'Brien J, Swann A, James I (2001b) *Treating Behavioural and Psychological Symptoms of Dementia*. Oxford University Press, Oxford

Ballard CG, Thomas A, Fossey J et al (2004) A 3-month randomized, placebo-controlled, neuroleptic discontinuation study in 100 people with dementia: the neuropsychiatric inventory median cutoff is a predictor of clinical outcome. *J Clin Psychiatry* **65**(1): 114–9

Birks JS, Harvey R (2004) Donepezil for dementia due to Alzheimer's disease (Cochrane Review). In: *The Cochrane Library*, Issue 2. John Wiley & Sons, Chichester

Brodaty H, Ames D, Snowdon J et al (2003) A randomized placebo-controlled trial of risperidone for the treatment of aggression, agitation, and psychosis of dementia. *J Clin Psychiatry* **64**(2): 134–43

Cohen-Mansfield J, Lipson S, Werner P et al (1999) Withdrawal of haloperidol, thioridazine, and lorazepam in the nursing home: a controlled, double-blind study. *Arch Intern Med* **159**(15): 1733–40

Committee on Safety of Medicines (2004) *Atypical antipsychotic drugs and stroke* (9 March) www.mca.gov.uk/aboutagency/regframework/csm/csmhomemain.htm

(accessed 25 May 2004)

Cummings JL, Tariot PN, Graham SM et al (2004) *Effect of memantine on behavioural outcomes in moderate to severe Alzheimer's disease.* Poster presented at the American Association for Geriatric Psychiatry, 17th Annual Meeting, Baltimore

De Deyn PP, Rabheru K, Rasmussen A et al (1999) A randomized trial of risperidone, placebo, and haloperidol for behavioural symptoms of dementia. *Neurology* **53**(Sep): 946–55

Douglas S, James I, Ballard C (2004) Non-pharmacological interventions in dementia. *Adv Psychiatr Treat* **10**(3): 171–9

Finkel SI, Costa e Silva J, Cohen G et al (1996) Behavioral and psychological signs and symptoms of dementia: a consensus statement on current knowledge and implications for research and treatment. *Int Psychogeriatr* **8**(suppl 3): 497–500

Howard R, Ballard C, O'Brien J, Burns A (2001) UK and Ireland Group for Optimization of Management in Dementia. Guidelines for the management of agitation in dementia. *Int J Geriatr Psychiatry* **16**(7): 714–7

Katz IR, Jeste DV, Mintzer JE et al (1999) Comparison of risperidone and placebo for psychosis and behavioral disturbances associated with dementia: a randomized, double-blind trial. Risperidone Study Group. *J Clin Psychiatry* **60**(2): 107–15

Lyketsos CG, DelCampo L, Steinberg M et al (2003) Treating depression in Alzheimer's disease: efficacy and safety of sertraline therapy, and the benefits of depression reduction: the DIADS. *Arch Gen Psychiatry* **60**(7): 737–46

Nyth AL, Gottfries CG (1990) The clinical efficacy of citalopram in treatment of emotional disturbances in dementia disorders. A Nordic multicentre study. *Br J Psychiatry* **157**(12): 894–901

Olin J, Schneider L (2004) Galantamine for Alzheimer's disease (Cochrane Review). In: *The Cochrane Library*, Issue 2. John Wiley & Sons, Chichester

Roth M, Mountjoy CQ, Amrein R (1996) Moclobemide in elderly patients with cognitive decline and depression: an international double-blind, placebo-controlled trial. *Br J Psychiatry* **16**(2): 149–57

Street JS, Clark WS, Gannon KS et al (2000) Olanzapine treatment of psychotic and behavioral symptoms in patients with Alzheimer disease in nursing care facilities: a double-blind, randomized, placebo-control-led trial. The HGEU Study Group. *Arch Gen Psychiatry* **57**(10): 968–76

Sultzer D, Gray KF, Guny I et al (1997) A double blind comparison of trazodone and haloperidol for the treatment of agitation in patients with dementia. *Am J Geriatr Psychiatry* **7**(1): 60–9

Tariot PN, Erb R, Podgorski CA et al (1998) Efficacy and tolerability of carbamazepine for agitation and aggression in dementia. *Am J Psychiatry* **155**(1): 54–61

Tariot PN, Jakimovich LJ, Erb R et al (1999) Withdrawal from controlled carbamazepine therapy followed by further carbamazepine treatment in patients with dementia. *J Clin Psychiatry* **60**(10): 684–9

Teri L, Logsdon RG, Peskind E et al (2000) Alzheimer's Disease Cooperative Study. Treatment of agitation in AD: a randomized, placebo-controlled clinical trial.

Neurology **55**(9): 1271–8

Wild R, Pettit T, Burns A (2004) Cholinesterase inhibitors for dementia with Lewy bodies (Cochrane Review). In: *The Cochrane Library*, Issue 2. John Wiley & Sons, Chichester

Key points

- Behavioural and psychological signs and symptoms of dementia (BPSD) are common and a major source of stress to family carers, often leading to long-term care.

- Some such symptoms will pass naturally or may not upset the person with dementia, and therefore do not need treatment.

- Psychosocial interventions should be considered and tried before drug management.

- A number of drugs may be useful for BPSD, but most will have side effects or lack a strong evidence base.

- The cholinesterase inhibitors may turn out to be more useful for BPSD than some of the alternatives.

- Depression should certainly be treated in dementia: this will sometimes involve antidepressants but may involve non-pharmacological treatments.

- Treatment should be rational, taking a broad view of the person, and should be reviewed.

Chapter 7

The environment and dementia: Shaping ourselves

Julian C Hughes, Debra Harris

We are all affected by our environments. Michael Manser (1997), an architect writing about environments for people with dementia, quoted Winston Churchill as saying, 'We shape our buildings, thereafter they shape us.' But our environments are not solely built; they are also constructed socially.

We shall go on to discuss both the social and the built environment. Before doing so, we shall consider delirium, which shows how the environment can worsen or ameliorate a person's confusion. Snoezelen, meanwhile, is an attempt to use the environment very specifically in a therapeutic way. But before looking at these specific examples of how the environment can be important, we should pause to consider the meaning of space and in particular, the personal meaning of space.

The phenomenology of space

The palliative care approach lays emphasis on the need to be holistic. In this book, we have understood this to mean that the person is a 'situated embodied agent' (Hughes, 2001). One of the ways in which we are inevitably situated is as embodied agents in space. In some sense, the space that surrounds us contributes to our standing as persons:

> *'Space is not just a geometric or mathematical construct that is objectively out there in the world. Rather, space is an aspect of human experience.' (Agich, 2003)*

Agich goes on to outline how in various ways, illness or disability alter the person's perception of the world. The environment of the person confined to a beanbag becomes severely limited:

> *'...not just de facto...but limited as an essential condition. For the elder requiring long-term care, confinement is an essential feature of existence.'*

As dementia worsens and the need for care increases, the person's perceived environment is likely to become more confusing and distressing. Just as the person's ability to cope with new things diminishes, there may be a new location and new carers to get to know.

Negotiating the new environment, which would be tricky for anyone, becomes much more difficult. The previous two chapters have discussed the psychological and pharmacological ways in which the confusion and distress that might result from worsening dementia can be dealt with. In a sense, this chapter points towards ways in which the confusion and distress might be prevented, or at least lessened, in the first place

The first step, if prevention is to be successful, is to see the importance of the individual's unique perception of space. There is no reason to think that the older person's perception will be vastly different from the younger person's. The older person going into long-term care would choose:

'...a location where life can be seen; an opportunity to see and mix with other age groups; a private place to live with your own possessions; and the choice to come and go and lead the life you like. A place to try to live in, not one to wait in to die.' (Manser, 1997)

The space surrounding the person with dementia needs to be one in which the individual can live as fully as possible:

'For people with dementia, familiar artefacts, activities and spaces can provide valuable personal associations and can stimulate opportunities for social interaction and meaningful activity.' (Cohen and Weisman, 1990)

Although the person's capacities to interact are diminishing, too often he or she is diminished as a person by the limitations of the social and physical space in which he or she must now exist. For,

'The sense of self is the sense of being located at a point in space, of having a perspective in time and of having a variety of positions in local moral orders...human beings become persons by acquiring a sense of self. But that can only occur in social milieu in which they are already treated as persons by others...' (Harré, 1993)

Social space

The adverse effects of the social environment are best (and now famously) summed up by Kitwood's (1997) phrase 'malignant social psychology'. Social

Table 7.1: Elements of malignant social psychology (Kitwood, 1997)	
• Treachery	• Banishment
• Disempowerment	• Objectification
• Infantilization	• Ignoring
• Intimidation	• Imposition
• Labelling	• Withholding
• Stigmatization	• Accusation
• Outpacing	• Disruption
• Invalidation	• Mockery
• Disparagement	

space is made up of verbal and non-verbal communications. Kitwood observed how easily personhood could be undermined in dementia by too little attention being paid to the need we all have for meaningful communication in a way that induces wellbeing, rather than illbeing. Kitwood's definition of personhood runs as follows:

'It is a standing or status that is bestowed upon one human being by others, in the context of relationship and social being.'

To be ignored, to be tricked into staying somewhere we do not wish to stay or to be talked down to, cause ill being and undermine the individual's standing as a person. Kitwood's full list of the elements of malignant social psychology are shown in *Table 7.1.* Kitwood (1997) states:

'The strong word "malignant" signifies something very harmful, symptomatic of a care environment that is deeply damaging to personhood, possibly even undermining physical wellbeing.'

He adds that 'malignant' does not imply evil intent on the part of care givers:

'The malignancy is part of our cultural inheritance.'

This led Kitwood and his colleagues in the Bradford Dementia Group to develop Dementia Care Mapping (DCM): an observational method intended to allow systematic recording of the nature of the interactions experienced by the person with dementia over an extended time. Crucially, the judgement about the nature of the experience must be made from the perspective of the person with dementia in order to ensure that the method is 'person-centred'.

DCM has so far stood the test of time and its use in various care settings and for research has increased worldwide (Ballard et al, 2002; Fossey et al,

Table 7.2: Features of delirium	
• Abrupt onset • Fluctuating global disorder of cognition • Impairment of consciousness and attention • Evidence of underlying physical precipitating factors	• Psychomotor disturbance • Disturbed sleep–wake cycle • Emotional upset • Perceptual problems: misinterpretations, illusions or hallucinations

2002), even if there are grounds for considering how the method might be improved (Beavis et al, 2002).

Confusion and the environment

The thought suggested by Kitwood's work is that the social environment might be enhancing, but might also add to the person's confusion and irritability. The person might not be able to recall, for instance, what has happened to him or her during the day, but he or she might be left with a sense of frustration and deep annoyance having been repeatedly disempowered, ignored, infantilized or tricked. One way to avoid irritability and aggression, therefore, might be to get the social environment right in the first place. The aim of DCM is to help this process.

But it is not just the social environment that counts. The physical environment also needs to be considered. Before discussing this in a little more detail, it is worth noting that environmental factors are seen as central to the management of delirium, i.e. acute confusion.

The deterioration in the behaviour of Mr Abode (see case study) needs to be explained. A sudden change in his behaviour might have a variety of causes. For instance, there may be features suggestive of depression. But the possibility of delirium needs to be taken seriously (*Table 7.2*).

Case study: Mr Abode

Mr Abode has severe dementia. He does not audibly speak and is reliant on staff for all his personal care. He has been in a nursing home for about 6 months. His pattern of behaviour has been settled: while awake, he wanders up and down the single corridor in the home, seemingly in his own world; he rarely sits. He is aggressive during personal interventions.

Over the last week he has started to hit on the fire door at the end of the corridor and he has become increasingly aggressive with staff when they try to intervene. When not hitting on the door, he has a greater tendency to drowsiness than usual. It is thought he might be hallucinating because he mumbles more and seems distracted. He becomes particularly agitated if he is in communal areas and there is noise from other residents; there are concerns he may become aggressive towards them.

The treatment of delirium, where there is a more or less sudden onset of confusion or increased confusion, is the treatment of the underlying condition. The causes of delirium are many and are listed in standard texts (Mulligan and Fairweather, 1997). Advice on management, although it usually includes the judicious use of medication to control disturbed behaviour as a last resort (see Chapter 3), always stresses the importance of the general environment:

> *'The nursing environment should be kept as quiet as possible,*
> *with minimization of extraneous noise from, say, television*
> *and radios, and noisy ward equipment such as pumps, alarms,*
> *and bleeps. Efforts should be made to provide visual cues for*
> *orientation such as clocks and calendars…the patients should*
> *be encouraged to wear their normal spectacles and hearing*
> *aids to increase awareness of the environment.' (Stewart and*
> *Fairweather, 2002)*

Patients with delirium need to be nursed in rooms with good lighting so that the tendency to misinterpret the environment is minimized. The atmosphere must be calm, again to decrease confusing sensory inputs.

It is worth remembering Mary Marshall's (2001) suggestion that, 'noise is as disabling to people with dementia as stairs are to people in wheelchairs.' In the case of delirium, therefore, both the physical and the social environments play a role in management. In some cases, patients with delirium may need to be transferred to a unit that is better able to provide an appropriate environment, but this will depend on a careful balancing of the benefits and risks posed by such a move.

The immediate use of psychotropic medication, which carries the risk of possible adverse effects, commonly reflects the pressure of time, the concerns of relatives and poor communication between different members of staff. Environmental interventions, which pose minimal risks, are often overlooked (Meagher, 2001).

It should be recalled that delirium is not uncommon in patients with dementia, especially as they become more frail, and it is not uncommon in people who are dying. Not only, therefore, must delirium be picked up, but it should be adequately managed as part of good quality palliative care in dementia (Goy and Ganzini, 2003). As we have seen, this will involve attention to the social and physical environment.

Sniff and doze

In Chapter 5, the use of multisensory environments was considered briefly. Kitwood recognized Snoezelen as a possible means to enrich the lives of people with dementia. It may be that people with dementia, like Mr Abode in the case study, can be helped to calm without the use of medication, but with regular use of Snoezelen.

Whereas interventions such as reality orientation and reminiscence are useful in meeting the needs of older people who can communicate, things appear more difficult for those who cannot. Relaxation, which might be one component of the management of Mr Abode's aggression, is particularly difficult because of sensory deficits and other impediments to communication, such as cognitive deficits. Sensory problems and cognitive decline, therefore, combine and contribute to the impoverished lives of people with dementia. Hope (1997) offered the suggestion that:

> *'Multisensory environments go some way to meeting these needs and improving quality of life for patients and carers'.*

Snoezelen is an amalgam of the Dutch words for 'sniff and doze'. It aims to stimulate the senses by combining soft lighting effects, tactile surfaces, meditative music and relaxing essential oils. There are many types of Snoezelen equipment; including lava lamps, bubble tubes, fibre optic strands and image projectors. Aroma diffusers are frequently used, along with background music for auditory stimulation. Kempenaar et al (2001) said:

> *'Providing appropriate and accessible stimulation can promote communication and wellbeing, by increasing sensory stimulation.'*

Social isolation can result because of the sufferer's increasing inability to form and sustain meaningful attachments with people. Snoezelen aims to improve staff–patient relationships by using an enabling approach. This needs to be used with sensitivity, flexibility, awareness and personal warmth.

Snoezelen encourages better quality relationships between staff and residents in homes simply by requiring that time is spent being with the person, rather than doing to, which may be particularly helpful in working with aggressive residents, since relationships may be strained or staff may feel demoralized. Dowling et al (1997) stated:

> *'The main long-term benefits for Snoezelen patients were in the area of socially disturbed behaviour.'*

Baker et al (1997) agreed:

'Patients in the Snoezelen room showed a significant decrease in socially disturbed behaviour and an improvement in mood.'

They suggested that Snoezelen is effective in preventing 'a pattern of dementia'.

Snoezelen seems to encourage relaxation in a helpful way (Schofield, 2000) and as such, it may be a useful adjunct to the control of pain. Pinkney (1997) discussed how the Snoezelen effect can reduce or eliminate intellectual demands as sensory experiences are unpatterned. This, and the enabling approach, helps patients to relax as fewer intellectual demands are made upon them (Baker et al, 1997). Verbal expression seems to be facilitated when the person's thoughts and responses do not have to be consciously organized.

A Cochrane review of Snoezelen in dementia (Chung et al, 2004) identified that it is commonly used therapeutically in dementia for four reasons:

- To reduce maladaptive behaviours and increase positive behaviours
- To promote positive mood and affect
- To facilitate interaction and communication
- To promote a caring relationship while reducing caregiver stress.

The same review could find only two trials (Baker et al, 1997; Kragt et al, 1997) that were randomized and controlled and in which Snoezelen or multisensory stimulation programmes were used as an intervention for people with dementia. The review concluded that there was not enough evidence to make positive recommendations about the use of Snoezelen in dementia care, even if one of the studies showed some trends in the direction of improvements in a number of areas. Nevertheless:

'From the practice perspective, Snoezelen programmes demonstrate positive immediate outcomes in reducing maladaptive behaviours and promoting positive behaviours, suggesting that it should be considered as part of the general dementia care programme. However, the limited carryover and long-term effects of Snoezelen programmes suggest that a continuous and ongoing programme should be implemented.' (Chung et al, 2004)

The shaped environment

As Hoskins and Marshall (2002) wisely remark, design is not everything, even if it is important:

Table 7.3: Designing for dementia (Marshall, 2001)	
Principles of design	**Design features**
• Compensate for disability	• Small size
• Maximize independence	• Domestic
• Enhance self-esteem and	• Allow ordinary activities
confidence	• Unobtrusive safety
• Care for staff	• Different rooms for
• Orientate	different functions
• Reinforce personal identity	• Age-appropriateness
• Be welcoming to all	• Safe outdoor space
• Allow control of stimuli	• Single big rooms
	• Good signs and orienting cues
	• Objects to orientate
	• Enhanced visual access
	• Controlled stimuli, especially noise

'Design will not address some issues such as low morale, poor skills, inadequate staff support, an unstimulating regime, and so on. Design makes good care easier. It does not make it happen.'

But the design of the buildings in which care is given is important, not only for the wellbeing of the people with dementia, but also for the staff and the families who look after them. The need for good design remains even as dementia worsens:

'During the later stages of dementia, patients become unaware of their surroundings. Until this point is reached, all the characteristics that make a good building easy to use by normal people become even more important and have to be developed to a new peak of clarity.'
(Manser, 1997)

Even if it is true that the person with severe dementia is less aware of his or her environment, there are still challenges for the designer who wishes to fit together a space suitable for the wandering of Mr Abode, with the complexity that surrounds the needs of people who are dying (Cox, 1996). Not only might dying people require equipment, such as hoists and special beds, but in the spirit of holistic terminal care, the space must be comfortable for their families.

In the context of dementia, Marshall (2001) suggests that there is a consensus around both the necessary principles and features of design (*Table 7.3*). The design must allow staff ready access to patients who might be anxious and restless; and similarly should allow the people with dementia to see other people, even if they do not wish to join in with activities (Hoskins and Marshall, 2002).

In the future, and increasingly already, design will include technology that allows people to be monitored throughout most of their daily routines (Demongeot et al, 2002). While contributing to safety, however, these advances also raise important ethical questions (Hughes and Campbell, 2003).

Many units now include circular pathways, which allow the wandering behaviour of Mr Abode to continue unabated. This seems better than the person constantly coming to a locked door, which will repeatedly cause frustration. Conversely, the constant circular wandering may simply be a way of adding to the person's disorientation. Mary Marshall (1997) states:

> *'I would argue that some of these people go on walking because they never get anywhere and they are in fact bewildered and lost.'*

Instead, it may be better if the wandering brings the person to somewhere that might seem familiar, to a lounge or kitchen, or through a garden to a different entrance and back to a communal area.

Finally, the design should allow space for the person's individuality. As the dementia worsens and the person's particular characteristics fade or become more inscrutable, his or her personal history will be held to some extent by the environment. The person will be held, not only by the memories of friends and family, but also by those personal artefacts that help to recall earlier times: the photograph of the picnic by the side of the road perhaps.

> *'Personal space provides the best means possible for orienting people to the person they were and still are. It is also important for staff, often part-time and relatively transient, to know about the people they are caring for. Single rooms should reflect the history and personality of the person.' (Marshall, 1997)*

Conclusion

In this chapter, we have considered the social and the built environments and the impacts they have on people with dementia, particularly as the person becomes more confused and must increasingly rely on the environment. Delirium is a good example of a situation in which the environment (social and physical) may contribute to the confusion, but may also be used to ameliorate the problem. Snoezelen offers a further example of how the environment might be used in a palliative way, to ease symptoms of irritability and anxiety in the more severe stages of dementia.

The central message, however, is the Kitwood message: the standing of the person as a person will be bolstered or undermined by the environment. We do not detract from the importance of the built environment by stressing the critical nature of the social environment.

Kitwood's message encourages the new culture of dementia care. It is a message that has been elegantly and forcefully conveyed in the writings of Steven Sabat over a number of years. We live in our environments, which in dementia become ever more restricted; but we are also 'positioned' in our environments, both physically and socially, in ways that either encourage or inhibit how we present ourselves:

'To assume that the afflicted person's social self is immune to the effects of how he or she is positioned by others would be to make a potentially grievous error and such an error would, in turn, make the process of caregiving far more difficult for everyone concerned.

'On the other hand, to cooperate with the afflicted in constructing valued social personae would mean, in principle, an easing of social isolation, the ability to continue and even develop rewarding relationships...in this way, the afflicted person's confinement would be determined more by the boundaries of neuropathology and less by the social misunderstanding which derives from innocently misguided positioning.' (Sabat, 2001)

References

Agich GJ (2003) *Dependence and Autonomy in Old Age: An Ethical Framework for Long-term Care*. Cambridge University Press, Cambridge: 136–43

Baker R, Dowling Z, Wareing LA, Dawson J, Assey J (1997) Snoezelen: its long-term and short-term effects on older people with dementia. Br J Occup Ther 60(5): 213–18

Ballard CG, O'Brien JT, Reichelt K, Perry EK (2002) Aromatherapy as a safe and effective treatment for the management of agitation in severe dementia: the results of a double-blind, placebo-controlled trial with Melissa. *J Clin Psychiatry* 63(7): 553–8

Beavis D, Simpson S, Graham I (2002) A literature review of dementia care mapping: methodological considerations and efficacy. J *Psychiatr Ment Health Nurs* 9(6): 725–36

Chung JCC, Lai CKY, Chung PMB, French HP (2004) Snoezelen for dementia. In: *The Cochrane Library*, Issue 2. John Wiley & Sons, Chichester

Cohen U, Weisman GD (1990) Environmental design to maximize autonomy for older adults with cognitive impairments. *Generations* **14**(suppl): 75–8

Cox S (1996) Quality care for the dying person with dementia. *J Dementia Care* **4** July/Aug: 19–20

Demongeot J, Virone G, Duchene F et al (2002) Multi-sensors acquisition, data fusion, knowledge mining and alarm triggering in health smart homes for elderly people. *C R Biol* **325**(6): 673–82

Dowling R, Baker R, Wareing LA, Assey A (1997) Lights, sounds and special effects. *J Dementia Care* **Jan/Feb**: 16–18

Fossey J, Lee L, Ballard C (2002) Dementia care mapping as a research tool for measuring quality of life in care settings: psychometric properties. *Int J Geriatr Psychiatry* **17**(11): 1064–70

Goy E, Ganzini L (2003) End-of-life care in geriatric psychiatry. *Clin Geriatr Med* **19**(4): 841–56, vii–viii

Harré R (1993) *Social Being*. Blackwell, Oxford: 4

Hope KW (1997) Using multi-sensory environments with older people with dementia. *J Adv Nurs* **25**(4): 780–5

Hoskins G, Marshall M (2002) Expect more: making a place for people with dementia. In: Jacoby R, Oppenhimer C (eds) *Psychiatry in the Elderly*. 3rd edn. Oxford University Press, Oxford: 460–83

Hughes JC (2001) Views of the person with dementia. *J Med Ethics* **27**(1): 86–91

Hughes J, Campbell G (2003) The electronic tagging and tracking debate. *Nurs Res Care* **5**(4): 174–7

Kempenaar L, McNamara C, Creaney B (2001) Sensory stimulation with carers in the community. *J Dementia Care* **Jan/Feb**: 16–17

Kitwood (1997) *Dementia Reconsidered: The Person Comes First*. Open University Press, Buckingham and Philadelphia

Kragt K, Holtkamp CCM, van Dongen MCJM et al (1997) [The effect of sensory stimulation in the sensory stimulation room on the well-being of demented elderly. A cross-over trial in residents of the R.C. Care Center Bernardus in Amsterdam]. *Verpleegkunde* **12**(4): 227–36

Manser M (1997) Better quality environments for people with dementia. Design of environments. In: Jacoby R, Oppenhimer C (eds) *Psychiatry in the Elderly*. 2nd edn. Oxford University Press, Oxford: 410–23

Marshall M (1997) Better quality environments for people with dementia. Design and technology for people with dementia. In: Jacoby R, Oppenhimer C (eds) *Psychiatry in the Elderly*. 2nd edn. Oxford University Press, Oxford: 424–35

Marshall M (2001) Care settings and the care environment. In: Cantley C (ed) *A Handbook of Dementia Care*. Open University Press, Buckingham and Philadelphia: 173–85

Meagher DJ (2001) Delirium: optimising management. *Br Med J* **322**(7279): 144–9

Mulligan I, Fairweather S (1997) Delirium – the geriatrician's perspective. In: Jacoby R, Oppenhimer C (eds) *Psychiatry in the Elderly*. 2nd edn. Oxford University Press, Oxford: 507–26

Pinkney L (1997) A comparison of the Snoezelen environment and a music relaxation group on the mood and behaviour of patients with senile dementia. *Br J Occup*

Ther **60**(5): 209–12

Sabat SR (2001) *The Experience of Alzheimer's Disease: Life Through a Tangled Veil*. Blackwell, Oxford: 308

Schofield PA (2000) The effects of Snoezelen on chronic pain. *Nurs Stand* **20**(15): 33–4

Stewart N, Fairweather S (2002) Delirium: the physician's perspective. In: Jacoby R, Oppenhimer C (eds) *Psychiatry in the Elderly*. 3rd edn. Oxford University Press, Oxford: 592–615

Key points

- The environment is crucial to the person with dementia.
- Confusion (in dementia and in delirium) can be ameliorated by the environment.
- The social environment can undermine or enhance personhood.
- The physical environment can frustrate or encourage good care.
- Snoezelen may contribute to good environmental care.

Chapter 8

Quality of life for people with dementia

Lynne Corner, Julian C Hughes

There is an ever increasing body of work on the quality of life of older people, including people with dementia and their carers (Bond and Corner, 2004). To date, however, less attention has been paid to quality of life at the end of life: that is, the quality of dying in dementia, an area which raises complex and controversial philosophical and moral issues.

Quality of life: A difficult concept

Quality of life is a term that is widely used, but one that is difficult to define. One problem is that there is little consensus over definitions and terminology and little agreement, for example, about what constitutes quality of life and what affects quality of life. From one perspective, quality of life is very subjective; what one person considers important to his or her quality of life will differ to what someone else thinks is important, and these opinions may change over time. It is its subjective nature that is particularly problematic to researchers and practitioners trying to assess a person's quality of life.

But, from another perspective, there are objective features that contribute to quality of life. Someone in considerable pain, for instance, or suffering from obvious mental distress, could hardly be said to be enjoying a good quality of life. Hence, a really accurate measure of quality of life would take account of both its subjective and objective aspects. This poses problems for measuring quality of life under any circumstances, but the problems are perhaps more keenly felt in dementia: not only is it difficult to agree on the objective features of quality of life, but also it seems increasingly impossible to know what would contribute to the person's subjective quality of life as dementia worsens.

This 'subjective–objective problem' is, however, not the only problem. There is also the 'problem of domains' and the 'problem of then and now' (Hughes, 2003). Before moving on to consider these problems, it is worth saying something about measurement in this field generally.

A big research industry exists to try and measure quality of life (Ready and Ott, 2003), but we may be trying to quantify a topic that is not always directly measurable. Depending on whose perspective you take, which is always a perspective at a certain point in time, you may wish to focus on different aspects of quality of life. So, for example, a psychiatrist may focus on the effects of a person's depression on his or her quality of life, a carer on his or her lack of social interaction. These aspects of quality of life, or features that contribute to quality of life, may be measurable for specific purposes.

But the concept of quality of life itself is simply too broad and deep to be measured. To measure something requires that it is bounded, but quality of life does not have clear boundaries because it is different for different people at different times. This is so even if particular aspects of quality of life, say the person's ability to be physically independent, can be measured for particular purposes.

Someone might object that we all make value judgements about a person's quality of life and, in fact, it is necessary that we should do in clinical practice in order to make the difficult decisions that have to be made. For example, there are difficult decisions about when it is appropriate to withdraw or withhold treatment that inevitably hinge, at least in part, on an assessment of the person's quality of life. But these value judgments are precisely that: they are evaluative judgements that bring into play all sorts of concerns.

> *'Once we see this, we realize that measurement is not the main concern, although it may have a role. Rather, we require understanding, listening, balancing, careful negotiation, empathy, along with attention to the needs and views of others who might be enmeshed with the person who is our concern.*
>
> *If this is an uncomfortable conclusion for the scientist, it should not be. For the realm of values and judgements about what makes our lives good or bad is the world that we normally inhabit.' (Hughes, 2003)*

Quality of life for older people

There is now a considerable amount of research identifying the domains that people of all ages consider to be important to their quality of life (Farquhar, 1995) and a more limited literature on the domains that older people consider important (Fry, 2000). The broad traditional domains identified in quality of life research with older people are highlighted in *Table 8.1*.

Generally, the factors that older people highlight are the same for other age groups. These broadly include: relationships with family and friends; social contacts; their own health, independence, mobility and ability; emotional wellbeing; material circumstances; religion or spirituality; leisure activities;

Table 8.1: Domains relevant to the quality of life of older people

Subjective satisfaction:
   Global quality of life as assessed by individual older person
Physical environmental factors:
   Standard of housing or institutional living arrangements, control over
   physical environment,access to facilities such as shops, public transport
   and leisure providers
Social environmental factors:
   Family and social networks and support, levels of recreational activity
   and contact with statutory and voluntary organizations
Socioeconomic factors:
   Income and wealth, nutrition and overall standard of living
Cultural factors:
   Age, gender, ethnic, religious and class background
Health status factors:
   Physical wellbeing, functional ability and mental health
Personality factors:
   Psychological wellbeing, morale, life satisfaction and happiness
Personal autonomy factors:
   Ability to make choices, exercise control and negotiate ownenvironment

and home environment (Farquhar, 1995). Issues such as social integration, the importance of having a purpose in life and belonging to a community have also been identified as hugely valued and central to people's understanding of their quality of life (Bamford and Bruce, 2000).

Other factors that are important to quality of life include self-esteem, a sense of self and identity, a sense of control and spiritual wellbeing. These concepts are important for people having a positive view of themselves and they impact on their relationships with friends, families and their activities. However, they have been largely ignored in the assessment of quality of life for older people in health care settings, which tends to focus narrowly on health issues.

But while this research into the domains of quality of life might make it seem as if the domains have some sort of concrete reality, of course they do not. The fact that many different researchers have identified similar domains, or domains that overlap, does not preclude the possibility that an individual may come up with something different that, nevertheless, contributes to his or her quality of life.

Contrariwise, the fact that different researchers come up with so many different accounts of the domains of quality of life might be taken as evidence that the domains cannot ultimately be pinned down. This is the 'problem of domains' that we referred to earlier.

One way to avoid the spectre of ever-multiplying domains would be to plump for very broad domains, by which every conceivable aspect of the good life might be subsumed. The problem then, however, is that the domains become increasingly difficult to measure for the reasons we mentioned above, namely that concepts as broad as 'health' (whether physical or mental) are notoriously difficult to pin down.

The perspective of older people with dementia

Improving or maintaining quality of life is surely the ultimate goal of all care and services for people with dementia and their carers. But how do we know what people with dementia are experiencing? What do older people with dementia and their carers consider important to their quality of life? How do they judge what is important to them and what they need? And what might be the best approach to evaluate quality of life for people with dementia?

Many clinicians and researchers argue that we cannot know what people with dementia experience because they cannot tell us. However, many people in the early stages of dementia can relate their feelings and experiences (Logsdon and Albert, 1999). Although the time taken to interact with people in the later stages of the disease may increase, there is research evidence that meaningful information can be obtained (Russell, 1996).

People with advanced dementia may not be able to tell us about their experiences using the same forms of expression as people without cognitive impairment (i.e. verbal communication), but this does not necessarily stop us from developing informed insights into what they are experiencing (Sabat and Harré, 1992). To begin to understand what is important to their quality of life requires time, patience and frequent contact.

Some progress has been made in assessing the quality of life of people with dementia in nursing and residential care using Dementia Care Mapping (DCM) (Kitwood, 1997). DCM was developed as a measure of quality of care, rather than quality of life. However, for people in long-term settings, the quality of care provided is perhaps most closely equated with higher levels of quality of life.

DCM has been used to illustrate that lower performance on activities of daily living and higher use of psychotropic medication in residential and nursing homes tends to have an adverse effect on quality of life (Ballard et al, 2001). Observational methods used in residential care settings have focused on residents' 'engagement', on the assumption that increased engagement or interaction is associated with better 'quality of life'.

Approaches using observational techniques have specifically focused on the quality of interactions between people with dementia (Perrin, 1997). However, such approaches to assessing quality of life remain in their infancy and are time-consuming and expensive. Research has tried to combine different approaches to ensure that the perspective of people with dementia is represented (Brod et al, 1999; Logsdon et al, 1999; Selai, 2001).

Individuals rarely operate in isolation and a person's life will consist of a rich biography of different relationships and experiences. People with dementia face many assaults on their quality of life, not just as a result of the disease process, but from the reactions of others to them. For example, they are frequently labelled as lacking insight and will consequently more acutely experience depersonalization (Kitwood, 1997), loss of independence, restriction of activities, loss of social and political rights and their behaviour being individualized (i.e. blamed on them and not ascribed to the disease), ultimately, of course, with a direct effect on their quality of life. The case of Bob and Mary illustrates some of these points.

Case study: Bob and Mary

Bob had always enjoyed running and for over 35 years he had been an active member of a local running club, training with fellow members for marathons and completing daily training runs. The running club also constituted a major part of his social life; he and fellow members met once a week in a local pub and he had developed many close friendships with other club members. Running was clearly important to his quality of life and to his sense of identity. He described the sense of freedom he had always felt when running, how he found running relaxing and how he cleared his mind, running on 'auto-pilot'. The sense of achievement he felt when completing a run was 'fantastic':

'Your body feels good all the time, that's what it feels like, it drives you on because you are wanting to do that all the time and get faster.'

This enthusiasm only came to light following a chance remark by his wife, when discussing 'days gone by'. When questioned about what was important to their quality of life, neither raised the topic. Bob had been experiencing memory problems for 6 years when he was diagnosed with probable Alzheimer's disease. Almost immediately following this diagnosis, Bob withdrew from running. Friends from the local club no longer contacted him to join them. This had been particularly hurtful to Bob and he had felt unable to contact his friends, and his closest friend in particular, for an explanation as to why the contact had ceased. Bob's wife Mary explained:

'...a friend of his, a very good friend actually, they've been running for years together, came out and saw him last year and said "Right Bob, I'm still running...I'll come and pick you up and I'll take you and I'll bring you back, give us a ring if you want to go". So, I says "Do you want to go?" "Yes". So I rang and told him he wanted to go and he never rang back and that really, really upset him. I don't think he ever got over that.'

Mary described the effect that this incident had had on Bob:

'I think he's frightened of getting let down again... he's frightened to trust again.'

Mary felt Bob could no longer go out running, focusing on the risks involved and the potential consequences. She expressed her fear of him being hurt and getting lost and unable to find his way home.

Bob no longer goes out running. He said that he wished he could still run, and felt that he still could. Physically, he remains fit and lean, with the body of an athlete, but restrictions have been placed by others on his choices. No attempt was actually made to facilitate him pursuing his enjoyment of running. For example, there is an enclosed park nearby. This was deemed by others as an 'unacceptable risk'. Professionals legitimized the carer's feelings and no attempts were made to take on board just how important running was to Bob's self-concept. This emphasis on the dementia and the losses had a huge effect on his quality of life, and a catastrophic effect on how he perceived himself.

Quality of life for people with advanced dementia

We now understand much more about the experience of dementia from the person's perspective. However, the methodological and theoretical challenges to understanding and assessing the quality of life of older people with very advanced dementia are immense. This group of people is often omitted from research studies, largely because of the challenges to verbal communication, with researchers opting to focus attention on people with the early or moderate stages of the disease process.

We know very little about what people with advanced dementia experience in the latter stages of the disease, and what gives their life quality, because they cannot tell us using conventional research methods. To date, then, less attention has been paid to the quality of a person's life at the end of life, or the quality of dying. Quality of life in the terminal phases of dementia will be a critical part of the study of quality of life in the future. Several scales have been developed to try and facilitate the measurement of quality of life in more advanced dementia (Albert and Logsdon, 2000). They tend to rely on proxy reports and do not involve the patient directly.

One way to involve the patient is to find out what he or she wishes before the dementia becomes too profound. Advance directives (or living wills) might allow clinicians some understanding of what might be important for the person. But, among other things, they raise the third problem we mentioned above: 'the problem of then and now'.

Advance directives and quality of life

There is a patchy literature on advanced directives in dementia and their use in end-stage dementia. Some of the ethical issues relating to advance directives have been touched upon in Chapter 4.

From the legal point of view, advance directives are properly thought of as advance refusals of treatment. That is, you can state what treatments you do not wish to have under particular circumstances. So, this only gives a rather limited insight into what constitutes quality of life for an individual. It has the potential, however, to emphasize to the clinical team that you are interested more in quality than in quantity of life, perhaps, although it does not say much about the more everyday aspects of care. For this reason, some people have advocated a broader advance statement of values that might well help carers to decide what the person would have regarded as the best course of action.

In addition, since dementia progresses from the day of diagnosis to the day of death, the change in the person caused by the dementia and by the label of 'being demented' is profound. Moreover, the person is likely to have made the advance directive some time before the dementia became apparent. This raises the 'then and now' problem. Then, when the advance directive was made, you might have regarded dementia as the thing most to dread; now, you may be content, despite having dementia.

Philosophers have raised this as a problem in deciding between the interests of the 'then self' and the 'now self'. One worry is that taking a rather stark objective view of quality of life in severe dementia could lead to a limited value being placed upon the lives of people affected by dementia. Bringing in some aspects of the 'then self' will help to give a broader picture of the person and may encourage attention to some of the key domains of quality of life, such as choice, control and dignity. However, to ignore how the person is now seems to undervalue his or her personhood (Jaworska, 1999).

Conclusion: Palliative care and quality of life

Given the problems with quality of life as a concept, what should be said of its central role in the philosophy of palliative care? We have already argued that it is a concept that can be used, even if it is not one that can be successfully measured. It is used in the broad context of everyday practice where values and facts rub shoulders. Part of its use is, of course, that it focuses our attention away from 'quantity' of life. It leads us to think of the broader concerns that dominate human life beyond the realms of clinical science.

In some ways, the other principles underpinning palliative care stem from this concern with 'quality'. Hence, we need to take into account the whole person; we need to pay attention not only to symptoms, but also to the person's psychological, social and spiritual problems; we need to encourage the person to live as fully as possible until death; we need to involve the person's family, friends and other carers. What this amounts to is a broad understanding of the person, which allows the problems of subjectivity and objectivity, of domains and of then and now, to be reconciled (Hughes, 2003).

Clearly, understanding more about quality of life in the terminal stages of dementia will be a critical part of future study, but that study will need to pay as much attention to conceptual and moral concerns as it does to empirical data (Jennings, 2000).

References

Albert SM, Logsdon RG (eds) (2000) *Assessing Quality of Life in Alzheimer's Disease*. Springer Publishing Company, New York

Ballard C, O'Brien J, James I et al (2001) Quality of life for people with dementia living in residential and nursing home care: the impact of performance on activities of daily living, behavioral and psychological symptoms, language skills, and psychotropic drugs. *Int Psychogeriatr* **13**(1): 93–106

Bamford C, Bruce E (2000) Defining the outcomes of community care: the perspectives of older people with dementia and their carers. *Ageing Soc* **20**(5): 543–70

Bond J, Corner L (2004) *Quality of Life and Older People*. Open University Press, Buckingham

Brod M, Stewart AL, Sands L, Walton P (1999) Conceptualization and measurement of quality of life in dementia: the Dementia Quality of Life Instrument (DQoL). *Gerontologist* **39**(1): 25–35

Farquhar M (1995) Elderly people's definitions of quality of life. *Soc Sci Med* **41**(10): 1439–46

Fry PS (2000) Whose quality of life is it anyway? Why not ask seniors to tell us about it? *Int J Aging Hum Dev* **50**(4): 361–83

Hughes JC (2003) Quality of life in dementia: an ethical and philosophical perspective. *Expert Rev Pharmacoeconomics Outcomes Res* **3**(5): 525–34

Jaworska A (1999) Respecting the margins of agency: Alzheimer's patients and the capacity to value. *Philos Public Aff* **28**: 105–38

Jennings B (2000) A life greater than the sum of its sensations: ethics, dementia, and the quality of life. In: Albert SM, Logsdon RG (eds) *Assessing Quality of Life in Alzheimer's Disease*. Springer Publishing Company, New York: 165–78

Kitwood T (1997) *Dementia Reconsidered: The Person Comes First*. Open University Press, Buckingham

Logsdon RG, Albert SM (1999) Assessing quality of life in Alzheimer's disease: conceptual and methodological issues. *J Men Health Aging* **5**(1): 3–6

Logsdon RG, Gibbons LE, McCurry SM, Teri L (1999) Quality of life in Alzheimer's disease: patient and caregiver reports. *J Ment Health Aging* **5**(1): 21–32

Perrin T (1997) The positive response schedule for severe dementia. *Aging Ment Health* **1**(2): 184–91

Ready RE, Ott BR (2003) *Quality of Life measures for dementia.* www.hqlo.com/content/1/1/11 (accessed 31 May 2003)

Russell CK (1996) Passion and heretics: meaning in life and quality of life of persons with dementia. *J Am Geriatr Soc* **44**(11): 1400–2

Sabat S, Harré R (1992) The construction and deconstruction of self in Alzheimer's disease. *Ageing Soc* **12**(4): 443–61

Selai C (2001) Assessing quality of life in dementia. *Med Care 39*(8): 753–5

Between 1999 and 2003, LC was an Alzheimer's Society Research Fellow engaged in research on quality of life in people with dementia, whilst based at the Centre for Health Services Research in Newcastle. She gratefully acknowledges the support of the Alzheimer's Society. JCH was generously supported by a Wellcome Trust short-term fellowship in bioethics in 2003 to carry out research into the conceptual basis of quality of life in dementia.

Key points

- Quality of life is a difficult concept to pin down and it raises ethical issues in its assessment.

- In an ultimate sense, measurement of quality of life is not possible, but evaluative judgements about people with severe dementia must sometimes be made.

- Such judgements require a broad view of people to incorporate aspects of their 'then selves' and their 'now selves'.

- The palliative care approach encourages such a broad view, bringing into play concern for all aspects of the self (e.g. physical, psychological, social, spiritual), as well as for the person's family, friends and carers.

Chapter 9

Difficult decisions for family carers at the end of life

Clive Baldwin

Family carers of people with dementia report facing difficult moral decisions throughout their time as carers. These difficulties range from day-to-day matters, such as the extent to which they need to take over tasks and make decisions, to more fundamental issues, such as placing a relative in residential care or opting for palliative care in preference to aggressive intervention.

None of these decisions is taken lightly and carers experience what can be called an 'ethical burden' in attempting to discern what is the right thing to do (Baldwin et al, 2004). The range of areas in which family carers experience ethical dilemmas is shown in *Figure 9.1*. Many of these areas may be associated with events at the end of life: for example, medication and treatment issues, communication and professional ethics, feeding issues, advance directives and dealings with family and friends. Some of these ethical issues have been discussed elsewhere in this book, especially in Chapter 4.

Primarily using the experience of a daughter caring for her mother as an illustrative example, the issues around the end of life and, in particular, the decision to opt for palliative rather than allopathic care are explored.

The case and other examples in this article come from a research study into the ethical issues facing family members caring for someone with dementia (Baldwin et al, 2005). While not focusing on palliative care per se, the responses from participants covered the range of experiences of caring for a relative with dementia, including end-of-life issues.

Decision making at the end of life

Despite the fact that many carers become well-informed about dementia and its progression, few it seems are well-prepared for having to make end-of-life decisions. Many carers feel supported by professionals in practical ways, but often feel alone and unsupported when it comes to making ethical decisions (Baldwin et al, 2004). The combination of distress, the pressure of time and conflicting feelings may increase their feelings of burden and aloneness,

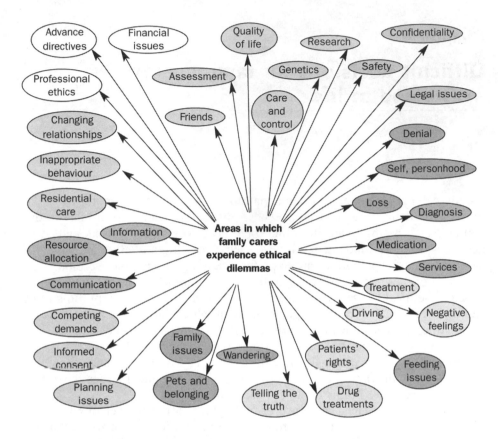

Figure 9.1: Typical ethical dilemmas

especially if in addition they feel that they have to fight over treatment decisions with professionals:

> '*So it was like...from the minute the hospital phoned I had a fight for a week with people – well it felt like that – and nobody taking decisions, and nobody helping you to make decisions or making stupid decisions!*' (*Daughter*)

Family carers and advance directives

Some carers think that if their relative had written an advance directive or living will as a means of providing some guidance as to his or her wishes, this would have alleviated some of the burden of decision making in difficult times. This view, however, is not universal and other carers are equally clear that advance directives can never foresee the complexities of future circumstances. According to this latter view, decisions about health and social care should be left to someone who knows the person well and has an emotional bond with that person.

In fact, very few carers reported that their relative had drawn up an advance directive or living will and only a handful reported that they had ever discussed end-of-life issues with their relatives. At present, in England and Wales, family carers are faced not only with making very difficult decisions with regard to their relatives, but also by a situation in which, until the *Mental Capacity Act 2005* (Stationery Office, 2005) comes into effect in 2007, there is no statute law underpinning their position as decision makers.

This is a significant disadvantage if they disagree with the health professionals involved in the care and treatment of their relative. In any disagreement with professionals, family carers may, in addition to feeling uncertain, anxious and possibly guilty, feel disadvantaged and unheard by those on whom they are relying to provide appropriate care and advice:

> *'We'd had a discussion in the morning about what was going to happen and we'd resolved, no more drips and she'd be nursed with oxygen and morphine if she got distressed. But she was written up for antibiotics intravenously because they'd forgotten to take it out of the medical chart.*

> *'So the nurse said, "Well, she's written up and I have to give her the drugs". And I said, "But we had this discussion earlier today that we weren't going to give it to her any more." So then they call a doctor and then she gets quite stroppy with us saying, "Well she's written up for antibiotics and it has to be intravenous and that means I have to put in a new drip."*

> *'So by this time we're at screaming point, because it feels all so unnecessary and that particular young doctor scrawled over the notes: "The relatives have refused to give her antibiotics".' (Daughter)*

Making decisions under pressure

In the absence of advance directives and discussions about end-of-life issues with their relatives, family carers are often faced with having to make serious decisions under the pressure of time and distress:

*'What happened when my mother got ill was that she went into hospital
and it was then fast decision-making time... While she was in casualty
she almost had a cardiac arrest so we were then saying, "OK, we're not
into reviving her", so you're making these quick decisions all the time,
you know. Yes, if the oxygen, you're going to help her breathe because
it's so distressing. Yes, if the antibiotics are going to make her breathe
better if she's not going to die. But if she's going to have a cardiac arrest
then no, we're not going to resuscitate her. And all these decisions were
made in the space of an hour while we were in casualty.' (Daughter)*

When faced with having to make decisions under such circumstances, carers
sometimes feel that they are swept along by the decisions of professionals:

*'I felt right at the very end maybe I should have said, "No you're not
going to move him." Maybe that was a decision I should have made
and I should have stuck with it, but at the time it just felt I was being
swept along with what they wanted.' (Wife)*

At such times, carers may ask themselves for whose benefit the decisions
are being made:

*'You could see by looking at my mother that you're not going to want
to resuscitate her, and I asked myself, "What's all this for, you know,
who is it for, all this stuff about antibiotics and drips and tissue?
You know, who is that for, whose benefit was it for? Was it for my
mother?" I don't think it was for my mother's benefit at all. It was to
make sure that you know the doctors had done their bit.' (Daughter)*

Differences of opinion as to what should be done are difficult for all
concerned. For the family carer, it is important that his or her relative be
allowed to die with dignity and this may mean without what he or she considers
to be undue intervention. As such, it is a decision made not only on the basis
of medical information and advice, but also one that is deeply rooted in carers'
emotions, life histories, values and relationships.

For professionals who do not share and may not even know the importance
of these factors in the decision-making processes of family carers, the decision
to intervene or not may be made primarily on the basis of medical evaluation
and prognosis. This is not to say that professionals override the wishes of
relatives out of arrogance or on a whim, but merely to recognize the fact that
their first duty as professionals is to ensure the wellbeing of their patients. As
our carer put it:

*'I think if you're into hospice care and palliative care, you understand
that there are other things that are important – but in an acute hospital,
the idea is that you do everything possible to prolong life.' (Daughter)*

Uncertainty

Decisions to forego potentially curative measures in favour of palliative care are not simple ones for family carers and invoke a great deal of uncertainty. This uncertainty arises from the tension between instinct and more rational consideration:

> *'The health issue has been very difficult because when someone is diagnosed with a life-threatening illness, your instincts say, "Let's try anything we can, any cure." But then I had to weigh up how much of the horrible treatments involved in lung cancer, how many of those treatments would he understand and appreciate and all of which would have been very frightening for him. But imagine, making that decision not to do anything except monitor and treat symptoms as they arose was really very difficult.' (Wife)*

Even when carers are certain in their own minds that the proper route is palliative care, it is not always clear to them where the boundaries lie between palliative and life-sustaining care:

> *'We decided we wouldn't artificially prolong my wife's life, but would treat symptoms that might be distressing. But even that's a fuzzy borderline because maybe the antibiotics we gave her for her urinary tract infection actually also protected her lungs as well. They might have done.*
>
> *'It was a long drawn out and very harrowing process and I actually wonder in retrospect whether that did her any favours, because there was no light at the end of this tunnel. It was just a tunnel that was going to go on into blackness. And I am still not clear as to whether it was actually in my wife's interests that she was maintained so long in this state.' (Husband)*

One carer reported that although she saw the reasoning behind the initial treatment on her relative's admission to hospital, she feared that instigating such treatment, rather than just palliative measures, would be the first step on a slippery slope to more aggressive and invasive treatments.

In their different ways, each of these carers experienced uncertainty in making their decisions about end-of-life care for their relative. Many carers express the feeling that after their relative died, they felt guilty that they had not done enough or the 'right thing' when their relative was alive:

> *'She slipped away peacefully. I was with her when she died and it couldn't have been more peaceful, which is a great relief to me. But*

after that comes the guilt. And this is very difficult to overcome.'

Such feelings of uncertainty and guilt may be particularly evident over decisions at the end of life.

The role of care home staff

Although many people with dementia die in hospital, this is not always the case and often they are cared for in residential or nursing homes. The staff in these homes may be in a strong position to offer support to family carers during the end stages of their relatives' lives.

Support for family carers with regard to end-of-life decision making perhaps starts with discussions when relatives are considering a placement in a residential or nursing home. Although family members may be reluctant to talk about end-of-life issues, many of them are concerned that their relative will not be unnecessarily moved from the home if or when their care needs increase. By discussing such issues with relatives, staff may be able to open up discussions about end-of-life issues at an early stage. Undertaking a 'values history' with both the person with dementia and family members may help prepare family members to make end-of-life decisions regarding their relative, should the time come (see www.unm. edu/~hsethics/valueshist.htm).

In contrast to acute hospital personnel, residential and nursing home staff often have contact with the person with dementia and family carers on a regular basis over a significant period of time. This contact facilitates the development of relationships and staff may come to know the values, desires, hopes, expectations and fears of family carers in a way and to an extent that could not be expected of acute hospital staff. Residential and nursing home staff are thus in a good position to advise and support family carers in an informed and sensitive way.

Carers may also be grateful for support by residential or nursing home staff in dealing with other professionals. In distressing times, it may be difficult for carers to think of everything they ought to ask or need to know:

> *'And sometimes, you know, you don't always ask the right question or the question that you think you've asked. Fortunately, on the day we had the discussion about continuing antibiotics, the deputy manager of the home was visiting us and said, "Do you want me to stay while you have this discussion?" Fortunately, she had the presence of mind to ask all the right questions, so that was really helpful.' (Daughter)*

Coda

Family carers, when faced with end-of-life decisions, feel disadvantaged. Not only are they being thrown into unfamiliar, difficult and emotionally painful situations, but they may also be uncertain of the legal force of their wishes and decisions. However, the passage of the *Mental Capacity Act 2005* (Stationery Office, 2005) helps to clarify the position in England and Wales. It establishes in statute law, not only the force of advance directives, but also the appointment of health care proxies or donees. A person appointed as such (the donee) will be able to make health and social care decisions on behalf of another (the donor), should the donor ever lack the capacity to make such decisions for him or herself.

Capacity legislation already exists in Scotland (Stationery Office, 2000). Although these measures should strengthen the position of family carers in the decision-making process, it is likely that carers will still require ethical and emotional support in making the difficult decisions that arise at the end of life. If staff in nursing and residential care homes have engaged with the person with dementia and his or her family, they will be well placed to give support to family carers making such decisions.

References

Baldwin C, Hope T, Hughes J, Jacoby R, Ziebland S (2004) Ethics and dementia: the experience of family carers. *Prog Neurol Psychiatry* **8**(5): 24–8

Baldwin C, Hope T, Hughes J, Jacoby R, Ziebland S (2005) *Making Difficult Decisions*. London: Alzheimer's Society.

Stationery Office (2000) *Adults With Incapacity (Scotland) Act*. The Stationery Office, Norwich

Stationery Office (2005) *Mental Capacity Act 2005*. The Stationery Office, Norwich

This research was undertaken at the Ethox Centre in Oxford. It was funded by the Alzheimer's Society under the Quality Research in Dementia programme. The views expressed are those of the author, but thanks are extended to the other members of the research team (Professor Tony Hope, Professor Robin Jacoby, Dr Julian Hughes and Sue Ziebland). Quotes are taken from interview transcripts and appear by permission of the participants.

Key points

- While carers may feel supported in practical ways by professionals, they often feel alone and isolated in making difficult ethical decisions.

- Few carers feel well prepared when they are faced by difficult end-of-life decisions regarding the care and treatment of their relatives.

- Care home staff are often in a strong position to support and advise family members because of their prior relationships with and knowledge of the person with dementia and his or her family.

- Even now that the position of family members in end-of-life decision making has been given a legal footing by capacity legislation, in England and Wales as previously in Scotland, it is likely that they will continue to need ethical support in making these decisions.

Chapter 10

When it's difficult to swallow: The role of the speech therapist

Jill Summersall, Sheila Wight

The primary role of the speech and language therapist (SLT) is the identification and treatment of communication disorders and swallowing difficulties. SLTs are increasingly involved, as part of the multidisciplinary team, in the diagnostic process during the early stages of dementia. They are also involved in the management of emerging communication difficulties, advising both clients and carers on strategies to aid successful communication. However, in the continuing care setting, the emphasis is largely on management of swallowing difficulties caused by the advanced nature of the dementia at this stage in the patient's care.

The involvement of the SLT usually begins with the initial signs of dysphagia (difficulty swallowing), such as reduced chewing or behavioural problems affecting eating. The incidence of dysphagia in dementia has been reported to involve as many as 93% of institutionalized elderly patients (Feinberg et al, 1992).

As the disease progresses to the advanced stages, it is often not possible to manage the dysphagia successfully without risk of aspiration, despite compensatory strategies. Patients are often immobile and are fully dependent for all care. Almost all patients, at this stage, have minimal or no language skills. It can be very difficult to achieve or maintain an optimum position for swallowing (Johnson and Scott, 1993).

Advancing cognitive impairment can result in behavioural problems such as vocalizing while eating. People with dementia have reduced awareness of food in their mouths and an inability both to chew and to swallow effectively. In addition, poor concentration and fluctuating consciousness place the resident at significant risk of aspirating food or liquids. Aspiration (entry of material into the airway below the true vocal cords) should be kept to a minimum to avoid the development of aspiration pneumonia (Logemann, 1983).

Rudman and Feller (1989) have highlighted how poor nutrition is a major contributor to a cycle of difficulty fighting infection. Christensson et al (1999) reported that protein-energy malnutrition in elderly people moving into residential care from the community or from hospitals was associated with higher morbidity, including pressure sores.

In the management of most neurological dysphagia, the next step, if aspiration were suspected, would be a video fluoroscopic investigation of

Table 10.1: Protocol management of dysphagia in advanced dementia

Patient referred for swallowing assessment, which results in one of three outcomes:

Level 1: Patients whose dysphagia can be satisfactorily managed
Disordered swallow that can be satisfactorily managed by dysphagia management strategies such as thickened liquids and positioning.
Protocol for Level 1 patients
- Swallow assessment completed, where possible with key nurse present.
- Written advice on swallowing regimen (patient-specific) provided to nursing staff/carers and consultants.
- Written advice should be displayed in nursing notes, on the whiteboard in the kitchen/dining room and in the patient's room, if appropriate.
- General leaflet on dysphagia in dementia given to relatives by key nurse.

Level 2: Patients who are at high risk of aspirating
Patient remains at high risk of aspirating despite introduction of dysphagia management strategies. For example: inability to position patient appropriately; patient continues to vocalize during oral intake; patient is unable to co-operate with management strategies; fluctuating alertness. Despite this, there are no overt signs of aspiration.
Protocol for Level 2 patients
- Swallow assessment completed, where possible with key nurse present.
- Written advice on swallowing regimen (patient-specific) provided to nursing staff/carers and consultants.
- Written advice should be displayed in nursing notes, on the whiteboard in the kitchen/ dining room and in the patient's room, if appropriate.
- Relatives informed of high risk of aspiration and its consequences by key nurse. Speech therapy leaflet on dysphagia in advanced dementia given to relatives by key nurse. This explains the likelihood that the swallowing problem will deteriorate and become life threatening.

Level 3: Patients who are aspirating
Despite introduction of conservative dysphagia management strategies, patient continues to display overt signs of aspiration such as:
- Coughing/choking during or immediately following oral intake
- Wet/gurgly voice quality during oral intake
- Respiratory distress/deteriorating chest status.
Protocol for Level 3 patients
- Swallow assessment completed, where possible with key nurse present
- Consultant will be contacted and advised that the patient is aspirating

---

- Team (consultant, speech therapist and key nurse) discuss management options, which include: either continue to give small amounts of pureed food and thick liquids orally, using maximum precautions; or implement palliative care – patient will be nil by mouth.
- Key nurse discusses management options with next of kin and provides leaflet on dysphagia in advanced dementia, where appropriate.

---

the swallow. If aspiration were found to be more than 10% of the bolus, despite other management strategies, non-oral feeding by nasogastric (NG) tube or percutaneous endoscopic gastrostomy (PEG) would be recommended. However, studies have shown that PEG or NG feeding is contraindicated in patients with advanced dementia. They are more likely to pull out the PEG tube (Frissoni et al, 1998), which may necessitate restraint.

PEG insertion has not been shown to stop weight loss in patients with dementia, nor to prevent malnutrition (Henderson et al, 1992). Tube feeding does not prevent the aspiration of oral secretions or the aspiration of refluxed gastric contents (Finucane et al, 1999). PEG insertion is a surgical intervention, which carries the risk of wound infection, peritonitis, haemorrhage and gastric prolapse, as well as the dangers of anaesthesia. In addition, hospitalization is a stressful experience for patients with dementia (Peck et al, 1990).

Changing practice

The types and patterns of referrals received from old age psychiatry continuing care wards in Newcastle upon Tyne fitted this picture in that a large majority were referrals for assessment of swallowing. In what follows, we shall consider how we have helped to change practice locally by the use of a protocol linked to training. The difficult issues around swallowing problems in dementia will emerge (see case studies below).

Case studies: Mrs X and Miss T

Mrs X had a diagnosis of multi-infarct dementia. Her swallowing had gradually deteriorated over the course of 2 years, from a normal diet and fluids to eating a soft diet only. Following a couple of small transient ischaemic attacks she was put on a pureed diet and thickened fluids. A careful review of the notes revealed a repeated history of chest infections, suggesting Mrs X had some silent aspiration of food and drink, which eventually built up and resulted in a chest infection. The patient was, therefore, Level 3 on the protocol discussed below (see *Table 10.1*).

Discussions with the team revealed Mrs X still derived immense enjoyment from food and drink, with no adverse symptoms such as coughing, choking or a gurgly voice. It was decided by the team to continue to feed her a pureed diet and thickened fluids, but her family was advised that aspiration was probably occurring and that she was at increased risk of chest infections.

Miss T's swallowing had gradually deteriorated, secondary to her Alzheimer's disease. On assessment of her swallowing, she was suspected to be aspirating on all textures, including pureed food and very thick liquids. This was despite maximum precautions, such as being fed very slowly by nursing staff with a teaspoon. Feeding resulted in coughing and some respiratory distress. In addition, there was facial grimacing and increased agitation. Nursing staff found it more and more distressing to feed Miss T, who then contracted a chest infection and became extremely unwell.

The team met to discuss the options. The chest infection had led to a further deterioration in her swallowing. In conjunction with her nieces (her closest family) it was decided, because of the distress oral intake was causing Miss T along with the obvious aspiration caused by a severely dysfunctional swallow, to stop oral intake and treat her palliatively.

Previous practice

There was no dedicated SLT service for patients with dementia. The community service was able to provide only one-off visits for assessment and advice.

Following assessment, the SLT advised the nursing staff on a range of measures, including diet and environmental modification, and also gave advice on feeding methods. This did not facilitate effective multidisciplinary communication between nurses and SLTs, particularly as these dysphagic patients tend to have complex and changing needs.

As the dementia reaches an advanced stage, residents may display a very wide variety of factors that can contribute to compromised swallowing. This requires a problem-solving approach to dysphagia management. Again, this was sometimes hard to achieve in a one-off visit, but in other cases nurses were very aware of what was required, but they had to wait for the SLT to visit and sanction the changes before they could be implemented.

Current practice

Funding was secured to provide five specialist SLT sessions a week in old age psychiatry. Following the recruitment of the current post-holders as specialists in dementia, it became possible to evaluate dysphagia services for both inpatient and continuing care nursing homes.

The following changes in practice were presented to both medical and nursing staff for consultation:

1. A revised swallowing protocol tailored to the needs of patients with dementia
2. A dysphagia nurse training package for senior nurses
3. Dysphagia awareness training for all staff involved in feeding patients
4. Improved dysphagia documentation.

The role of multidisciplinary team members is important in all dysphagia management. It becomes essential in the palliative care of residents with complex dysphagia in advanced dementia. The goal of multidisciplinary team working is essential to maintain an adequate level of nutrition and hydration while limiting the occurrence of aspiration. It was hoped these new developments would lead to improved multidisciplinary working.

Owing to the severity of dysphagia in advanced dementia, therefore, management proves very complex and requires different treatment protocols. Existing dysphagia protocols neither encompassed the issues raised when non-oral feeding methods (such as PEG and NG tubes) were not a management option, nor did they consider the ethical dilemmas this raised. These ethical issues are further discussed in the commentary that follows.

A dysphagia protocol for dementia

In our area, we devised a new protocol which was then agreed with nursing and medical staff (*Table 10.1*). According to the new protocol, following assessment, patients are graded into three levels of severity:

- *Level 1* – Patients whose dysphagia can be satisfactorily managed by strategies such as modifying diet, correct positioning or feeding strategies.
- *Level 2* – Patients who continue to be at high risk of possible aspiration because of factors such as continual vocalization during feeding or fluctuating alertness. These risks remain, despite introduction of dysphagia management strategies as above. These patients are graded Level 2 and the risks associated with aspiration are discussed with their relatives. This proves to be a significant proportion of the residents in the old age psychiatry continuing care homes in Newcastle.
- *Level 3* – As the disease progresses, some patients develop overt or chronic signs of aspiration, despite all management options. These signs may include recurrent chest infections, coughing or choking, 'wet' or

'gurgly' voice or respiratory distress when being fed. These patients are then identified as Level 3. The protocol prescribes that all management options will be discussed with the consultant, next of kin, nursing staff and SLT. Each case is examined individually by the team, taking into account a range of factors. A decision is then made whether to continue or withdraw oral intake.

The factors that may be pertinent could include whether or not the patient shows pleasure or distress when being fed, the quality of life the patient currently has and any views he or she may have expressed prior to his or her illness. The protocol ensures that each patient's individual circumstances will be considered. Prior to the introduction of the protocol, nursing staff often felt they were left to make these difficult ethical decisions.

Training needs

As a result of joint working with nurses to develop the protocol, a number of issues regarding skill mix were identified. Nurses in continuing care often had extensive practical dysphagia expertise. However, their understanding of the rationale for these management decisions was limited.

Although nurses had a good grasp of complex feeding regimens, this knowledge was often acquired only on an individual basis. Nurses were not expected to share this expertise in the form of written care plans with colleagues, since SLTs had responsibility for dysphagia assessment and management. Therefore, much of this information was not available to bank staff or staff who were unfamiliar with the patient.

The nursing staff had no recognition by the Trust of this specialist dysphagia knowledge. There were no identified guidelines regarding decision-making in dysphagia management. All changes to diet textures and thickener had to be authorized by the SLT. Often, this led to significant delays before patients were assessed.

The Health Advisory Service (1999) have stated that:

*'...increased availability of staff who have received specific training
to perform swallowing assessments across all days of the week, is
now a matter of urgency.'*

A nurse dysphagia training programme was already established on old age medicine wards and it had resulted in an increase in dysphagia awareness. Ward managers in old age psychiatry were asked to identify suitably qualified and interested nurses to train in old age psychiatry settings. It was felt that nurses should be of E grade or above to ensure they had significant seniority to influence changes to clinical practice, but were not solely involved in management.

Two nurses were identified from each inpatient ward and continuing care home to attend the training, which involved 2 days of theory followed by practical training. There were three sessions of assessment and management planning for a dysphagic client. Initially, the nurse observed the therapist. This was followed by a joint decision-making assessment. Finally, the nurse was observed by the SLT completing an assessment alone and making recommendations.

A series of swallowing awareness workshops were offered to all grades of nursing staff. Increased awareness of symptoms of dysphagia and practical training in the use of thickening agents has resulted in a reduction in the amount of thickener used. Patients are therefore less likely to become dehydrated (see below).

Residents often need to be fed. The skills of the nursing staff when feeding are therefore paramount. Studies have found that being dependent for feeding was the most significant risk when predicting factors in aspiration pneumonia (Langmore et al, 1998). During training, nursing staff were instructed to feed each other too quickly or too slowly. This reinforced the importance of following the dysphagia care plan recommendations!

New dysphagia documentation

New documentation has ensured better communication of recommendations using printed dysphagia care plans and patient-specific feeding instructions on whiteboards in dining rooms. Leaflets have been devised to inform relatives of the stages of dysphagia and its consequences. The leaflets have been provided from the onset of swallowing difficulties to ensure relatives are informed of the impact of dysphagia now and as the disease progresses.

All grades of nursing staff have increased awareness of symptoms of dysphagia and senior staff are now equipped with the best techniques to alleviate them. The SLT no longer deals with day-to-day management changes and acts instead as a consultant. Thus, the SLT can respond more quickly when complex cases arise and the nursing staff require additional expertise. The dysphagia nurse training and the revised dysphagia protocols have helped both nurses and SLTs to recognize each others' knowledge and skills and to work more effectively together.

Discussion

In the early stages of dementia many techniques such as food texture changes, the right environmental modification and advice on feeding methods can manage dysphagia very successfully. A patient with increased impulsivity may over-fill his or her mouth, which can create a choking risk, particularly with textures such as bread.

Appropriate supervision by nursing staff, who are aware of practical techniques such as cutting bread into small squares and ensuring the patient is only given one piece at a time, allows the patient to continue to enjoy eating safely. This can prevent over-conservative management, such as moving the patient onto a pureed diet too quickly.

Some patients may develop limb dyspraxia, which results in an inability to feed themselves using cutlery. However, if the patient is fed finger foods they are often able to retain the ability to feed themselves, which in itself makes swallowing likely to be safer for longer (Langmore et al, 1998).

Thickener is often required to prevent aspiration. In early dementia, very small amounts of thickener in drinks are sufficient to slow down the speed of the liquid bolus and allow fluids to be taken safely and still be pleasant to drink. However, untrained staff were more likely to over-thicken drinks, which can lead to dehydration since the patients often find them unpalatable. Training of staff ensured more accurate measurement and, therefore, reduced the risk of dehydration.

The training described in this article equipped nursing staff with relevant knowledge. This is now often successfully used without the need to refer to speech and language therapy. Nursing staff have reported improvements in the overall knowledge of dysphagia on the wards and in continuing care, along with a feeling of clinical satisfaction gained from the autonomy provided by their new role. It is now possible to provide patients with an appropriate and safe diet and fluid regimen without any delay.

References

Christensson L, Unosson M, Ek AC (1999) Malnutrition in elderly people newly admitted to a community resident home. *J Nutr Health Aging* **3**(3): 133–9

Feinberg MJ, Ekberg O, Segall L, Tully J (1992) Deglutition in elderly patients with dementia: findings of videofluroscopy evaluation and impacton staging and management. *Radiology* **183**(3): 811–14

Finucane TE, Christmas C, Travis K (1999) Tube feeding in patients with advanced dementia. *JAMA* **282**(14): 1365–70

Frissoni GB, Franzoni S, Bellelli G et al (1998) Overcoming eating difficulties in the severely demented. In: Volicer L, Hurley A (eds) *Hospice Care for Patients with Advanced Progressive Dementia*. Springer, New York: 48–67

Health Advisory Service (1999) *Not Because They Are Old: An Independent Inquiry into the Care of Older People on Acute Wards in General Hospitals*. Health Advisory Service, London

Henderson CT, Trumbore LS, Mobarhan S et al (1992) Prolonged tube feeding in
   long-term care: nutritional status and clinical outcomes. *J Am Coll Nutr* **11**(3):
   309–25

Johnson H, Scott A (1993) *A Practical Approach to Saliva Control*. Psychological
   Corporation, Oxford

Langmore SE, Terpenning MS, Schork A et al (1998) Predictors of aspiration
   pneumonia: how important is dysphagia? *Dysphagia* **13**(2): 69–81

Logemann JA (1983) *Evaluation and Treatment of Swallowing Disorders*. College
   Hill Press, San Diego

Peck A, Cohen CE, Mulvihill MN (1990) Long term enteral feeding of aged demented
   nursing home patients. *J Am Geriatr Soc* **38**(11): 1195–8

Rudman D, Feller AG (1989) Protein-calorie undernutrition in the nursing home. *J
   Am Geriatr Soc* **37**(2): 173–83

Key points

- Dysphagia becomes more problematic and common as dementia worsens.

- Members of the multidisciplinary team can become involved in basic assessments
  of swallowing and in tailored interventions in order to free speech and language
  therapists for more complex dysphagia management.

- Multidisciplinary involvement is required, along with the involvement of the family,
  when difficult decisions have to be made about treatment near the end of life.

- These decisions are clinical and ethical: they need to take a broad view of what
  might be best for the person concerned.

Ethical commentary

Julian C Hughes

The concern about artificial nutrition and hydration, which emerges in this
discussion of swallowing problems in dementia, is not uncommon. We have
already come across it in the case of Ernie in Chapter 2. Nutrition and hydration
raise significant physical problems in terminal care, as we saw in Chapter 3; and
the ethical issues were touched upon in Chapter 4. However, further specific
comment would seem to be warranted.

One approach to the ethical debate is to look at the consequences of the
proposed treatment. On the basis of the evidence that artificial feeding (using
NG or PEG tubes) does no good in severe dementia and may do harm (Finucane
et al, 1999), Gillick (2000) has argued that gastrostomy tubes should not be used
in advanced dementia. Similar conclusions follow from the application of the

principles of medical ethics (Gillon, 1986; and see Chapter 4): not only is there evidence that artificial feeding does no good (it is not beneficent), but it also does harm (it is maleficent). Furthermore, Gillick (2000) cites studies showing that most competent older people in a nursing home would not wish to have a feeding tube if they were unable to eat because of permanent brain damage. The proportion of people against feeding tubes goes up when they are told that they might need to be restrained to keep the feeding tube in place. Thus, for most people (but importantly not for all), if we are to respect their prior autonomous wishes, we should avoid feeding tubes. Finally, the principle of justice might be taken to suggest that, given the doubts about efficacy, the resources associated with (e.g.) the placement and use of a PEG tube would be better used to provide other aspects of palliative care to people with severe dementia.

And yet, there is an understandable, genuine and important worry about withholding food and fluid from patients. (The legal debate typically concerns whether or not artificial nutrition and hydration amount to a 'medical treatment'; but while a legal determination is relevant to the ethical debate, the underlying moral question, 'Is it a good or bad thing to withdraw or withhold food and fluid from someone?' remains – whatever the answer to the legal question.) According to the protocol described in this chapter (*Table 10.1*), for patients on Level 3 one management option would be that the patient would be 'nil by mouth'. The ethical concern is that this might mean we are starving and dehydrating our patients to death. Recall that in Chapter 3, Regnard and Huntley stated: 'The reality is that stopping nutrition and hydration too soon does not result in a rapid deterioration but in prolonged discomfort'.

The key judgement here may be over what is 'too soon'. In an interesting discussion of the Jewish tradition, Gillick (2001) makes a distinction between a person being a goses (a moribund person) and regarding people as treifah (where the person is in an incurable state from which he or she will 'surely die'). She argues that, where the person has severe dementia and is unable to eat, he or she should be regarded as dying and, she says, 'Nutrition and hydration administered via a feeding tube are no more natural and necessary than is oxygen via a ventilator' (Gillick, 2001). Her argument is based on three facts: first that the person's life expectancy is less than a year; secondly, that the person is suffering; but, thirdly, that the person would not suffer from feelings of thirst or hunger. She supplies evidence to support these premises.

Gillick's (2001) argument might be contested. My main qualms would be, first, that it is not always obvious that the person in advanced dementia is suffering in the ways suggested (i.e. there may be suffering we are just not attuned to). Secondly, if the person would otherwise live for up to a year, I would feel uneasy with the thought that I had brought about his or her death so early, especially given the comment from Regnard and Huntley in Chapter 3. This would just seem to me to be 'too soon' to let the person die from lack of food and drink. Does this mean, however, that no rational justification can be given for allowing people to die as Gillick suggests?

My response would be to urge that the whole context must be taken into consideration (Hughes, 2002). Once the person really is close to death – and the distinction between goses and treifah is interesting here, because it shows the need for a fine clinical and ethical judgement – to allow that process to go ahead, rather than try to prevent it, is to accept the reality of the human condition. This seems to have been the case with Miss T in the case study. If, alternatively, the person would otherwise probably survive some time, my inclination would be (as in the case of Mrs X) to continue to give small amounts of appropriately prepared food and drink in a careful way. There would have to be an acceptance that this in itself might hasten death by causing aspiration, but it would still seem to be a matter of good care to persevere with feeding as long as possible. In any event, the decision about what might be in the 'best interests' of the person would have to be taken broadly, bearing in mind that this should not be a decision purely about best medical interests (see *Table 3.7* in Chapter 3). These decisions are made in concrete circumstances and should involve all concerned.

The point to emphasize is that judgements about treifah must mean that the person is truly close to death before it becomes ethically unproblematic to withhold food and fluids. And a final caveat: all of this only applies to swallowing problems that form part and parcel (as it were) of dementia. Other causes of dysphagia, which might be either transient or amenable to various forms of treatment, raise different (but related) issues.

References

Finucane TE, Christmas C, Travis K (1999) Tube feeding in patients with advanced dementia. *JAMA* **282**(14): 1365 – 1370

Gillick MR (2000) Rethinking the role of tube feeding in patients with advanced dementia. *N Engl J Med* **342**(3): 206-10

Gillick MR (2001) Artificial nutrition and hydration in the patient with advanced dementia: is withholding treatment compatible with traditional Judaism? *J Med Ethics* **27**(1): 12-15.

Gillon R (1986) *Philosophical Medical Ethics*. John Wiley & Sons, Chichester.

Hughes JC (2002) Ethics and the psychiatry of old age. In: Jacoby R, Oppenheimer C (eds) *Psychiatry in the Elderly*. 3rd edn. Oxford University Press, Oxford: 863-95

Chapter 11

General practice perspectives: Co-ordinating end-of-life care

Julian C Hughes, Louise Robinson

Standard 2 of the *National Service Framework for Older People* (Department of Health, 2001) stresses the need for patient choice, integrated and co-ordinated services and support for carers. In the section on dementia (standard 7), there is neither mention of how care for people with advanced dementia should be provided, nor how patient choice in this difficult situation should be ensured.

It would be very reasonable to argue that it is the family GP who is best placed to ensure the integrated and co-ordinated approach, which is true to the wishes of the person with dementia, and which also meets the demands of the family.

While the GP remains involved throughout the course of the person's dementia, the involvement is perhaps more apparent at the beginning and again at the end. It is the GP who must first pick up the symptoms and signs of dementia. The evidence is that 40% of GPs are reluctant to diagnose dementia early (Audit Commission, 2002), with the consequence that referral to services and agencies, which might prove helpful to either the person with dementia or the family carers, is made late.

In this article, however, we shall be concentrating on the end of the person's life. Nevertheless, as we shall suggest, getting things right at the end might depend upon getting them right at the beginning.

Where people die

Just over 40% of people with dementia die in nursing or residential care (McCarthy et al, 1997). We have no real idea about the quality of dying for people with dementia in long-term care.

A recent American study of people with dementia admitted to a geriatric ward found that over 60% of them died with high levels of suffering (Aminoff and Adunsky, 2004). It might be that those admitted to hospital are in a worse state physically than those who die in residential and nursing homes, but the evidence is not encouraging. It suggests that people dying from dementia have symptoms and health-care needs comparable with cancer patients (McCarthy et al, 1997). While many people with cancer die in hospices, the number dying from dementia at present in the UK in hospices is negligible.

One model, to improve the quality of dying in dementia, would be for people with dementia to be looked after in a hospice or hospice environment. Specialist units for people with dementia who are in the terminal phase of their condition have been in existence, with some success, in the USA for some while. These units certainly help to encourage good terminal care in dementia by limiting unnecessary interventions, and they even decrease costs (Volicer et al, 1994).

However, it can be questioned whether this model is the most appropriate for the large numbers of people with dementia who do not require hospital care. Would they not be better off being cared for in their own homes, or in the institutions that have become their homes? Perhaps our aim should be to improve the care of people dying with or from dementia where they actually are: in nursing and residential care homes. And, on a day-to-day basis, it is GPs who mainly provide medical care in these settings.

Barriers to good quality primary care

What are the barriers to GPs and other primary health-care workers (such as district nurses) providing good quality care to people with advanced dementia in nursing and residential settings? There are three main related areas of difficulty: communication, organization (systems) and education (specialist knowledge and skill) (*Figure 11.1*).

Communication

First, communication is the cornerstone of good general practice. Ahead of most other branches of medicine, GPs have been aware for many years of the importance of the therapeutic relationship and of the extent to which this is, in itself, a means of treatment (Balint, 2000).

This is challenged, however, in the context of dementia – especially when it is advanced. Even if the GP has previously known the patient, communication can be particularly difficult in advanced dementia. Moreover, the reality is that the GP looking after residents in a particular home will not have known them before their arrival.

Patients with advanced dementia in nursing homes, for instance, have often passed through a hospital ward before being 'placed' in the available home,

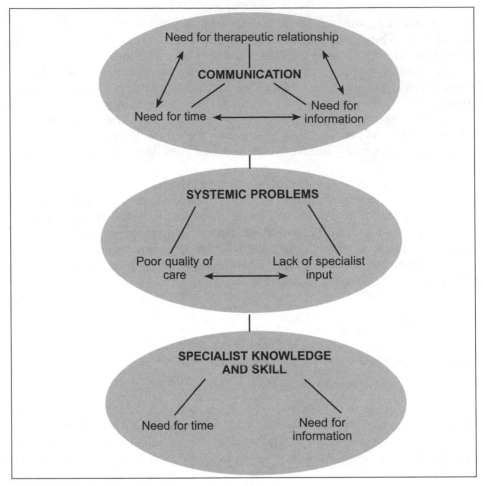

Figure 11.1: Barriers to good quality care in severe dementia

which may be some distance from where they previously lived. Unless the GP had been in regular contact with the person with dementia throughout the course of the illness, it would be difficult for a meaningful therapeutic relationship to be maintained.

A further difficulty from the point of view of communication is that the GP may lack the required time (Turner et al, 2004). Not only does this hamper getting to know the patient, but it also means that communication with family carers (who probably know more than anyone about the person's history, problems, inclinations and beliefs) is often minimal until a crisis is reached, when communication becomes vital, but also pressured (as described in Chapter 9).

Largely, the GP must rely on information from the staff of the home. Sometimes this will be very dependable, where the staff have known the person with dementia for some time, but it can be that staff are temporary, with only a scanty knowledge of the person concerned. Or, perhaps the care staff know the person, but are not familiar with the significance of the symptoms and signs he or she might be presenting. Thus, signs of a delirium on top of dementia might be misinterpreted as difficult behaviour, rather than as an acute event needing perhaps fairly simple remedial treatment. The possibility of a 'malignant' social environment is ever present (Kitwood, 1997; and see also Chapter 7).

Systemic problems

This leads us to the second type of barrier to good quality primary care for people with dementia. Systemic problems stem from organizational structures that affect the ways in which people relate and work.

In discussing communication, we have already gestured at problems associated with poor quality care for people with advanced dementia, but these problems are profound (Ballard et al, 2001). At a mundane level, the GP is likely only to see patients whom the staff highlight as requiring attention. At a deeper level, even when the GP perceives more general problems concerning the quality of care (for example, little activity or interaction for residents), it may not seem possible to change the culture within a home.

This sort of systemic problem is not one that solely faces GPs. As Professor Mary Marshall (2001) has noted, it is a staffing problem, but not one that can be fixed by blaming the staff. There are deeper problems, of which home managers will be acutely aware, to do with pay and conditions, retention of staff, motivation and understanding. The GP may feel him or herself to be one cog in a machine that does not produce the end product everyone would hope for, namely good quality care for people with advanced dementia.

Having said this, there are examples of good practice and dementia care mapping (Kitwood, 1997) provides one method to reflect critically on practice with a view to improving the quality of care provided to individuals.

Specialist knowledge and skill

The other problem facing GPs is that they may lack the specialist knowledge to intervene and improve standards (Turner et al, 2004). The Audit Commission (2002) certainly found evidence of limited specialist support: it was not available at all in 40% of all areas; and specialist services were not always adequately staffed.

Individual GPs may have the knowledge and skill base to advise on terminal care when the person is clearly dying. But the other types of problem that arise are the behavioural and psychological signs in dementia (BPSD) and this may be an area of unfamiliarity.

BPSD may occur in up to 90% of patients at some stage (Ballard and O'Brien, 1999). The recommended management is psychosocial (Douglas et al, 2004), but this can be a slow and painstaking process. So, it is no wonder that many people exhibiting such signs have found themselves on psychotropic medication, with all its deleterious effects (Ballard and O'Brien, 1999; and see Chapter 6).

Having knowledge and skill in both 'terminal' care and in the management of BPSD, both of which would form part of palliative care in dementia, would be a tall order for an individual GP without specialist support. However, it should also be acknowledged that the evidence base for any particular approach to agitated behaviour in dementia is thin.

Specialist knowledge usually involves an awareness of the breadth of treatment options, which often require trial on an empirical basis. The level of certainty that a particular approach will work is usually low and often it would be better to do nothing. The management of aggression requires an interpretation of the person's distress. Does it reflect pain or an emotional disorder? Is it an unavoidable consequence of a deteriorating brain? Or is it a consequence of the social environment? Building up expertise in this field is difficult.

This takes us straight back to systemic barriers to good quality care for people with advanced dementia. First, there is no overarching palliative care service for people with dementia that might provide both terminal care and management of BPSD. Second, specialist palliative care services themselves have tended to focus on cancer care: very few people with dementia receive hospice care, although the needs of cancer patients and dementia patients and their carers are probably similar (McCarthy et al, 1997).

This might seem to take us back to the idea of specialist palliative care dementia units, but (while acknowledging their utility) we have already discussed problems with such units, not least of which is the problem of deciding when the person has entered the 'terminal' phase (Schonwetter et al, 2003). Then, however, it can be questioned whether a move is in the person's best interests, rather than care in the community where the person actually lives.

Third, those who care for people with dementia in the community may feel they lack palliative care skills and those with palliative care skills can feel out of their depth dealing with people with dementia who exhibit BPSD (Evers et al, 2002).

Challenges

Having identified the barriers to good quality care for people with advanced dementia, how might they be challenged? We shall discuss four possible challenges (continuity of care, advance planning, the needs of carers and the need for specialist support) and then consider how such challenges might be mounted.

Continuity of care

How can continuity of care be provided, given the reality of the pathways taken by people with advanced dementia? In the ideal scenario, the GP would be involved with the family from before the diagnosis of dementia until the last stages. This would allow the GP to draw upon previous knowledge and accumulated trust to make the difficult decisions that might need to be made when the disease progresses.

This idealistic vision gets round problems with communication, it presumes that the quality of care in nursing and residential homes is good and that there is adequate specialist support. Hence, as we have seen, it is the ideal and not the reality. But it does demonstrate how some of the problems, mostly those around communication, might be circumvented by continuity of care.

Advance planning

We started by saying that one way to get the end right was to get the beginning right. If the diagnosis can be made at an early stage, the person with dementia would be in a position to discuss – in an empathetic environment – the issues that might arise in the future. This could be drawn up into an advance statement, expressing views and values, or (more legalistically) into an advance refusal of treatment.

It would also allow an increased understanding on the part of formal and informal carers concerning what might be in the person's best interests. Again, therefore, this would be a way to get round the barriers of communication in advanced dementia.

Needs of carers

One of the main tenets of palliative care is that a holistic view should be taken to include the views and concerns of the person's family. We know that many of the difficult decisions facing family carers occur as dementia worsens (see Chapter 9). They need to be included in discussions at an early stage. Moreover, they require support throughout the illness.

Preliminary evidence suggests that people with dementia and their carers appreciate a palliative care approach, which is not just confined to 'terminal' care (Shega et al, 2003). The carers of people with dementia often have to endure prolonged bouts of stress and strain. They develop their own patterns of bereavement, for instance, which are different from those experienced by carers of people with cancer (Albinsson and Strang, 2003).

It might be that the right support at the right time would help to alleviate some of the problems associated with advanced dementia. For instance, it might be possible to delay moves into long-term care. The barriers to good quality care are challenged both by involving carers early and by supporting them at home.

Specialist support

If specialist support were realistically available – to GPs, to nursing and residential homes, to family carers – it might be possible, by education and support to carers and to homes, to raise the quality of care for people with advanced dementia. It would need to involve specialists dealing with BPSD and with terminal care. There would need to be flexibility.

In addition, the existence of more specialist care might help to encourage research and improve the knowledge and skills base in this difficult area.

Mounting the challenge

Challenging the barriers to good quality palliative care for people with advanced dementia in the community is not a simple matter of admonishing GPs and specialists to do better, just as there is no point in blaming those who work in nursing and residential homes. We need something new.

This is not to say that we have to start from scratch. As this book amply demonstrates, the requisite knowledge and experience is to hand, but it is put into effect in a poor and patchy way, if at all.

The challenge should be mounted by teams that regard themselves as specializing in the treatment of advanced dementia. Such teams would, by their nature, be providing palliative care. In this context, palliative care must be understood to incorporate terminal care and the management of BPSD; and the care itself must be broad: person-centred but holistic, with an emphasis on psychosocial approaches, in addition to biological treatments, and with the involvement of the person's family and caring environment.

These teams would need to engage with people with advanced dementia where they are: not just in hospitals, but also in the community, in their own homes or in long-term care. As in the case of Macmillan nurses for cancer, these specialist teams must be in close contact with primary care. They might actually be based in GP units, or they might be based within revitalized NHS continuing care units for people with severe dementia.

The revitalization would entail such units no longer regarding themselves as the rump of the back wards of the old asylums. Nor would they be glorified nursing homes. In some places they have focused on 'challenging behaviour', which can be a helpful development. However, the notion of 'challenging' is ambiguous (challenging to whom?) and it leaves out the possibility of a broader view.

If they were to be considered as palliative care units for people with advanced dementia, dealing with BPSD (not just 'challenging behaviour', but apathy, depression and pain among other things) and providing a 'terminal' service, with in-patient beds, but also with outreach teams involving nurses with specialist skills in both palliative and dementia care, along with the full resources of a multidisciplinary team, their esteem would surely grow. They would be in a position to improve communication, encourage higher standards of care and increase specialist knowledge.

By becoming involved at an early stage, in conjunction with the GP, they could help to ensure continuity of care, facilitate advance care planning and consider the needs of the carers along with the needs of the person with dementia.

Conclusion

Sachs et al (2004), writing for general internists in America (akin to trainees in general practice), find similar barriers to those described above to good end-of-life care for patients with dementia. The understanding that dementia is a terminal illness is important for advance planning and from the perspective of Medicare (part of the insurance system, which dictates when hospice care is allowable).

They also highlight issues around communication, caregiving and bereavement. The ways around the barriers involve issues affecting public policy, education and better clinical practice. In large part what this means is a palliative care approach with appropriate symptom control and attention to the whole person. The benefits and the rationale for such an approach need to be understood by doctors, but also by patients, carers and the public.

Central to the implementation of good clinical practice in this field will be the GP. We have argued that the GP must be supported by a multidisciplinary, community-focused, person-centred, holistically-biased, specialist palliative dementia care team.

References

Albinsson L, Strang P (2003) Differences in supporting families of dementia patients and cancer patients: a palliative perspective. *Palliat Med* **17**: 359–67

Aminoff BZ, Adunsky A (2004) Dying dementia patients: too much suffering, too little palliation. *Am J Alz Dis Other Dem* **19**(4): 243–7

Audit Commission (2002) *Forget Me Not 2002*. Audit Commission, London.

Balint M (2000) *The Doctor, His Patient and the Illness*. Churchill Livingstone, Edinburgh

Ballard C, O'Brien J (1999) Treating behavioural and psychological signs in Alzheimer's disease. *Br Med J* **319**(7305): 138–9

Ballard C, Fossey J, Chithramohan R et al (2001) Quality of care in private sector and NHS facilities for people with dementia: cross sectional survey. *Br Med J* **323**(7310): 426–7

Department of Health (2001) *National Service Framework for Older People*. Department of Health, London

Douglas S, James I, Ballard C (2004) Non-pharmacological interventions in dementia. *Advanc Psychiatr Treat* **10**: 171–7

Evers MM, Purohit D, Perl D et al (2002) Palliative and aggressive end-of-life care for patients with dementia. *Psychiatr Serv* **53**: 609–13

Kitwood T (1997) *Dementia Reconsidered: The Person Comes First*. Open University Press, Buckingham

Marshall M (2001) The challenge of looking after people with dementia. *Br Med J* **323**(7310): 410–11

McCarthy M, Addington-Hall J, Altmann D (1997) The experience of dying with dementia: a retrospective study. *Int J Geriatr Psychiatry* **12**(3): 404–9

Sachs GA, Shega JW, Cox-Hayley D (2004) Barriers to excellent end-of-life care for patients with dementia. *J Gen Intern Med* **19**(10): 1057–63

Schonwetter RS, Han B, Small BJ et al (2003) Predictors of six-month survival among patients with dementia: an evaluation of hospice Medicare guidelines. *Am J Hosp Palliat Care* **20**: 105–13

Shega JW, Levin A, Hougham GW et al (2003) Palliative Excellence in Alzheimer Care Efforts (PEACE): a program description. *J Palliat Med* **6**: 315–20

Turner S, Iliffe S, Downs M et al (2004) General practitioners' knowledge, confidence and attitudes in the diagnosis and management of dementia. *Age Ageing* **33**(5): 461–7

Volicer L, Collard A, Hurley A et al (1994) Impact of special care unit for patients with advanced Alzheimer's disease on patients' discomfort and costs. *J Am Geriatr Soc* **42**: 597–603

Key points

- The GP is best placed to coordinate good quality end-of-life care for people with advanced dementia.

- The barriers to good quality care for people with advanced dementia include difficulties to do with communication, organizational systems and a lack of specialist knowledge and skill.

■ The barriers will be overcome by ensuring some form of continuity of care, by advance care planning, by including carers within the focus of care and by providing specialist knowledge and advice along broadly conceived palliative lines, to include the management of behavioural and psychological signs in dementia as well as terminal care.

■ The palliative dementia teams will need to be flexible, multidisciplinary and involved in the community, while also able to build up knowledge and skill through research and clinical experience.

Chapter 12

The spiritual care of people with severe dementia

Leslie Dinning

The most profound and often asked question, 'Why?', is not answered by me. I am unable to answer it. This is about my journey of learning and sharing, of just being there, of listening and of giving support. It is written from the viewpoint of the whole person and it approaches spiritual and pastoral care holistically. It sees the sufferer as a whole person, even though he or she experiences many losses during the illness.

Starting points

Offering spiritual care to a person can mean many things. But when the person has severe dementia, do we somehow clip the spiritual and offer an excuse or platitude because he or she is slowly withdrawing from life and changing? 'He does not know', 'She doesn't understand', 'Why bother?'. Such attitudes mask the fuller picture of the person's spirituality.

In the spiritual care of the sufferer of severe dementia, we must still see the whole person. This means that the chaplain has to get alongside and join in that person's journey and build up the picture. The chaplain meets sufferers when they are ill and probably have been for some time. It is now that we begin the journey with the person, the family and the staff and to engage with the sufferer's spirituality.

The theology of suffering is deep. It asks many searching questions but has no easy answers. Suffering caused by dementia can last a long time, causing carers and families to ask the deepest questions. These questions are often directed with anger at God, at staff, at the chaplain or at anybody to hand.

Christians may find hope in the suffering, death and resurrection of Jesus and express it through their spirituality. But what of those people who profess to have no faith? Where is their hope?

This is not a theological quest for answers to suffering. It is a story of spirituality, of seeing the whole person even through suffering. It is a story about spiritual wholeness in the depths of suffering. It is a story about being

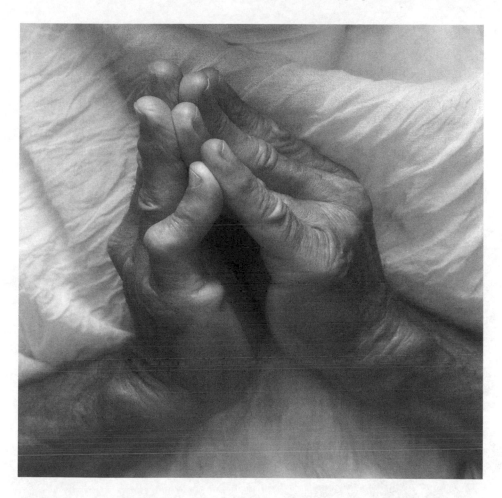

there and viewing the daylight, even if it has become narrow. It is about listening to stories as the family remembers the past with all its joys and emotions. It is also about the present.

When the daylight narrows

The journey has begun. It is not a journey we would plan – it just happens. It can be a slow journey into a place where the full daylight has become narrow. It shines into the room but does not light it up as once it did. It is in the shadows of suffering that we have to find the spiritual.

In any spiritual journey, the daylight has never gone. It is all too easy to make the judgement, because someone has lost speech and the ability to recognize people or places, or because he or she presents in a very different way to how he or she used to, that the person has lost everything. 'Why bother with spirituality?' I believe that the daylight, even though it is narrow, is still shining into the room of dementia. It gives hope.

Many people wait, not for a clear outcome but for a journey of uncertainty: uncertain where they are going or indeed where they may be taken. Life's transitional periods are characterized by uncertain change: the early years of parenthood, ill health, unemployment, retirement, redundancy, separation, divorce or bereavement. Donald Edie (1999) calls those in these states 'Saturday people'. They are people who, in a wide variety of circumstances, are learning the meaning of waiting during periods of sustained and wondering transition. As Edie says:

> *'There is a long Saturday between the Friday of crucifixion and the Sunday of resurrection.'*

The pain and distress of those who suffer, the long watch and wait of carers and of their families as the daylight narrows – the long Saturday of dementia seems never-ending. In this situation, I must meet the spiritual needs of the person with dementia. In doing so, I must also meet the needs of the family. It is a time for the spiritual care to begin by seeing the whole person in full daylight.

From full daylight (the past)

My first encounter with the dementia sufferer is on his or her admission to the assessment or to the continuing care unit. I then begin to get to know the resident. The staff are wonderful at introducing me and giving me some background information. After getting to know the resident and meeting the family, I have the opportunity to join in their spiritual journey. A relationship of trust has to begin.

It is about listening to the person's past, where he or she was born, the joys of courtship, of marriage and of family life: children, grandchildren and great grandchildren. He or she may have served in the Second World War. I hear of working life and of retirement. Or, perhaps, I hear the anger of the spouse because the retirement years have been taken from the person by the illness. There are stories told of hobbies, of holidays, of favourite songs and music, of the shared good and bad times. The full daylight has brought much into their lives and it forms part of the spiritual story, which we all share to some degree.

Some will tell how their spirituality has been expressed through a particular faith: their place of worship, the services they attended together, their involvement in different groups connected to their faith. Others will tell of how, as they grew older, they just drifted away from their faith. Still, they may remember its observances and traditions with affection.

All of this is very important for me in building up a picture of the person with dementia (see case studies). It is that person's identity and spirituality.

Case studies: Mrs A and Mrs B

Mrs A was cared for in a continuing care setting. Sometime before the onset of dementia she had been the victim of a violent and unprovoked attack. Initially, she could be found on fine days out and about in the grounds with members of her family or with the staff. She responded to a wave and a smile. As time went on, Mrs A's condition deteriorated and became more challenging. Her family were regular visitors.

One day, when walking past her room, I saw Mrs A sitting on the floor with her husband. He looked upset, and I asked after them both. He was keen to tell me that it was their wedding anniversary. The occasion was both spiritual and emotional.

Mrs B visited her husband in the nursing home every day without fail, arriving mid-morning and leaving mid-afternoon. This was a way of life for her. On a fine day, she would take her husband out for a run in the car or take him in his wheelchair into the grounds or the surrounding streets, stopping for an ice-cream or just sitting and enjoying the weather.

Early on in my conversations with Mrs B, I learned that both she and her husband had been regular worshippers at their local church. My offer to bring them both Communion on a monthly basis was taken up. This was always an emotional time for Mrs B as she remembered the Sunday mornings going to church with her husband and their walks on a Sunday afternoon.

We always had Communion in Mr B's room in the nursing home, surrounded by familiar photographs and ornaments. Mrs B always placed the Communion wafer into her husband's mouth. As he deteriorated, because of his difficulty swallowing, Mrs B suggested that perhaps Communion should stop. After a discussion, we decided to continue for a while longer with Mr B receiving only half of the Communion wafer.

The narrow daylight shines on the present

It is the glint of the narrow daylight shining through that makes the darkness and the dark places visible as the journey into dementia advances. The chaplain, in offering spiritual and pastoral support to the sufferer, has also to offer the same support to the family.

The majority of people suffering dementia will have been cared for in the early stages by their spouse at home. This involves the most intimate of tasks. On admission into the hospital, the carer's main role has been taken away. This brings a great sense of guilt: guilt that the person with dementia is no longer at home, guilt that the carer can no longer care for his or her loved one, guilt that the most intimate of tasks in caring are now done by someone else.

With guilt comes anger. This can be directed towards the staff, who are now the carers. They may complain about anything and nothing, often becoming vocal about the way their partner is dressed, the food that is offered or the room being unsuitable. This is, I believe, the spirituality of emotion and feelings.

The chaplain is not immune from these emotions. God seems to take the blame:

'He is a cruel God if He allows this to happen.'

'There is no God at all.'

'How can you believe in a loving God when He allows this to happen?'

'You would not let a dog suffer like this.'

Others will put their whole trust in God, by faith and prayer and the support of the chaplain and their local church or faith group. This helps them through. For them it is not about questioning God. It is about letting God share the journey with them.

Spiritual and pastoral care has to be about letting the carers and families have time and space to be angry, to show emotion and to voice how it really is for them. Even the God of suffering, death and resurrection lets people have time and space to ask the deep and hurtful questions that dementia brings. If God did not allow people to do this, then where would we begin to find the theology of suffering? People will always need safe and confidential spaces. The chaplain, as a spiritual caregiver, has to offer this for all, including the staff.

It is important to make carers realize that they have not been shut out of their caring role. It has not been taken away from them. They are encouraged to visit regularly, even at mealtimes, when they can help. They can join in social events and take part in the carers' group. They remain involved by being consulted on the person's likes and dislikes, favourite food or clothing and how often the hairdresser should call. Personalizing the room with pictures, photographs and ornaments and bringing in the person's favourite music and songs are all aids to remembering and creating a homely and friendly environment.

Again, I believe this is spiritual care performed as part of the overall care of the person.

The narrow daylight begins to fade

As dementia progresses, the changes in a person can be both frightening and dramatic. The changes in character, behaviour and communication can be very difficult for the family, as can the loss of recognition, the immobility and the weight loss. The person has journeyed from full daylight to narrow daylight and now the light is fading. This is not the person the family members have known all their lives:

'I lost him when the illness began.'

Some families have great difficulty in visiting because of the changes brought on by dementia. They may visit for a short time or the visits become increasingly infrequent. They become too emotional. Some families live too far away. The reaction of their neighbours and friends can be helpful or hurtful. Some will offer support, others will ask questions, such as 'Why do you go and visit so often when he doesn't even know you?' or 'Why don't you go and have a holiday? She won't miss you'. It is difficult for families to explain their need to be there for their loved ones.

The spirituality of love, care and devotion does not come to an end because a partner has developed dementia. Caring for someone with dementia is embracing the spirituality of life. It is remembering the past with the present. It is still seeing something of hope in the fading light. It is about sharing, joining in. It is the spirituality of wholeness.

This can be of some help and comfort at the end of a visit: travelling home alone, entering an empty house that is still full of memories, facing another night alone in fear of the telephone ringing – it might be the nursing home. Waking the next morning, it all begins again.

The narrow daylight shows the tears (end of life)

If we are viewing the dementia sufferer as a whole person and caring for his or her spiritual needs, we must also look at the spirituality that comes with the end of life.

The journey into dementia can last for many years. It is during this time that members of the sufferer's family have experienced many losses, many small bereavements. They have experienced the living deaths, such as the loss of recognition, of communication, of companionship. Perhaps the greatest loss of all is watching someone change from the person they have known and loved for years.

Yes, death comes to us all. When loved ones have watched someone slowly die over a long period of time, his or her death is often seen as a blessed release. Death becomes the welcome healer, for it has brought the suffering to an end.

The spirituality of the whole person must also include the spirituality of end-of-life issues. Watching a loved one who has suffered from dementia for many years will often bring family members to a discussion of what to do at the end of the sufferer's life. It gives them the opportunity to plan the rite of passage. As a chaplain called to a bedside to offer prayers and support for the sufferers and their family, I often find myself drawn into these discussions. These are very spiritual moments for us all. Families and staff need time and space to talk and explore these issues.

Spirituality at the end of life is often expressed through religious belief. Prayers are asked because 'He used to go to Church' or 'She has always believed in God'. As a chaplain, I am only too happy to be available for residents and their families at this time. Conversations around death and the planning of the funeral are very profound for us all. God, faith and religion are discussed in depth. The words and prayers of the Christian burial or cremation service, for instance, can be important in our understanding of great suffering and in the search for meaning.

It is also possible for the partner of the sufferer of dementia to die first. Families may or may not want the resident told. Wanting the person with dementia to know his or her loved one has died demonstrates a positive attitude towards the illness and the sufferer's understanding of events. In my experience, many families wish to be inclusive in this way. Will the sufferer be able to attend the funeral service? If not, families have asked me to hold a service in the home after the funeral, the invitation being extended to the staff too. The service would normally contain the words of the funeral service and an explanation at each stage of the service. Family members read the messages of condolence from the cards, and flowers are placed in the room.

I well remember Mrs C, a sufferer of dementia who attended her husband's funeral service – she smiled gently throughout. Even though the daylight becomes narrow, it does bring with it a ray of sunshine in the most painful of moments.

The spiritual care of the whole person has to include the spirituality of death and dying. When a person has suffered for a long period of time with dementia, death is seen as the great healer – for death brings peace. A great sense of relief is often felt. The planning of the funeral as a celebration and thanksgiving of life is also a very real part of the spiritual journey for the family. It is the last practical thing in which the family can participate.

Has the spirituality of the deceased died as well? I believe not, as it lives on in the memories held.

Conclusion

The chaplain's role in the spiritual care of people with severe dementia is a varied role. Spiritual care is offered at its best by nursing staff, clinicians, families and chaplains working together. I believe my role is 'being there'. It is being invited to share a very special spiritual journey.

The chaplain joins the journey when the daylight has become narrow. The chaplain's role is active and reactive. It means not just representing God in difficult situations; it also means trying to find God in the shadows when the full light has narrowed (see, for example, the story of Ellen below). The narrow daylight must never stop us seeing the whole person, for it is the spirituality of the whole person we are caring for.

> *'The spirituality of those who care for the dying must be the spirituality of the companion, of the friend who walks alongside, helping, sharing and sometimes just sitting empty handed, when he would rather run away. It is the spirituality of presence, of being alongside, watchful, available, of being there.' (Cassidy, 1988)*

This is what the spiritual caregiver is about: travelling the journey with the sufferer and his or her family and those who care for the person. We join the sufferer's spiritual journey. Let me end by reworking an old saying:

> *'There in the grace of God go they.'*

References

Cassidy S (1988) *Sharing the Darkness: The Spirituality of Caring*. Darton, Longman & Todd, London

Edie D (1999) *Grain in Winter: Reflections for Saturday People*. Epworth Press, Norwich

An introductory reading list and an annotated bibliography on the subject of dementia and spirituality have been produced by the Christian Council on Ageing Dementia Group. For copies, or details of the work of the Group, contact Alison Johnson, 33 The Plain, Brailsford, Ashbourne, Derbyshire DE6 3BZ. Tel: 01335 360591.

This chapter has mainly been written from a Christian perspective. An alternative resource with multi-faith contacts is: The Levenson Centre for the study of Ageing, Spirituality and Social Policy, Temple Balsall, Knowle, Solihull, West Midlands, BN3 0AN, website http://rps.gn.apc.org/levenson/study.htm

Key points

- The chaplain's role is to be with people who are suffering; to support them and their families and those who care for them.

- Taking care of the whole person, which involves the multidisciplinary team, also means attending to his or her spiritual needs – a central plank in the philosophy of palliative care.

- As part of the team, the chaplain is there to help to bring to mind all that the person was and still is in the context of family and community.

- For some, spirituality is expressed through religious belief.

- Religious acts of worship can help the individual with dementia to maintain and express his or her personhood and can comfort and support family and friends through bereavement.

Ellen's prayer

Audrey Ball

Ellen had Alzheimer's disease. I met her when she was a resident on a continuing care unit for people with severe dementia. Her daughter had asked me to visit her mother on a regular basis to give her Holy Communion. She wished to keep her mother aware of things for as long as possible and in touch with all the regular events that made up her daily life until she became ill.

Ellen was a gentle, smiling woman with a deep sense of peace about her. She was deeply loved by her family. We established quite a beautiful friendship and routine. I would visit her on the ward and we would go into a quiet room to talk and pray, and Ellen would receive the sacrament. I would always say, 'Shall we say a prayer now?' and her reply was always the same: 'That's the best.' She would join in with familiar prayers as much or as little as she wanted to on the day. As her illness progressed, Ellen could no longer receive the sacrament and was often distracted and fidgety. I continued to visit her and we went for short walks indoors, always ending up in the quiet room. We would sit and hold hands for a while and then I would say, 'Shall we say a prayer now?' 'That's the best', she never failed to reply. On a day I shall never forget and before I could start a prayer, Ellen, in her gentle way, said her own prayer:

> 'Dear God, You are all that matters,
> Help us to be happy,
> Help us to be welcoming,
> We need each other.'

When Ellen died, at the Mass of celebration and thanksgiving for her life, her prayer was prayed. May she rest in peace.

Index

J

M

N

O

P

Q

R

S